Praise for *The Nurse Manager's Guide to Innovative Staffing,* Third Edition

"Staffing continues to be one of the most challenging aspects of the nurse manager's role. This book provides a comprehensive overview of staffing, from budgeting to scheduling, daily staff adjustments, and data analytics. It serves as a wonderful resource for both practical approaches and innovation in nurse staffing."

–Marla J. Weston, PhD, RN, FAAN
CEO, Weston Consulting, LLC
Past CEO, American Nurses Association

"These two authors have developed an amazing book that will fulfill two major purposes: an orientation guide for new nurse managers and a refresher for experienced nurse manager as they ponder the staffing implications of a new model of care. It is designed as a comprehensive, educational, thought-provoking toolkit with pertinent questions to help guide the nurse manager as they develop their staffing plans. Congrats to Dr. Mensik and Brienne Sandow!"

–Rhonda Anderson, DNSc(h), MPA, RN, FAAN, LFACHE, FACHT
Consultant/Surveyor, Global Healthcare Accreditation

"This remarkable book sets the standard for leading practices with staffing and scheduling. The core of nurse retention is staff engagement and well-being. These chapters provide practical guidelines to create excellent outcomes. This book should be required reading for anyone involved in these processes."

–Karlene M. Kerfoot, PhD, RN, FAAN
Chief Nursing Officer, Symplr

the NURSE MANAGER'S GUIDE to INNOVATIVE STAFFING

3rd ED.

Jennifer Mensik Kennedy, PhD, MBA, RN, NEA-BC, FAAN

Brienne Sandow, MSN, RN, NEA-BC

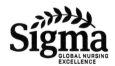

Sigma
GLOBAL NURSING EXCELLENCE

Sigma Theta Tau International Honor Society of Nursing (Sigma) is a nonprofit organization whose mission is developing nurse leaders anywhere to improve healthcare everywhere. Founded in 1922, Sigma has more than 135,000 active members in over 100 countries and territories. Members include practicing nurses, instructors, researchers, policymakers, entrepreneurs, and others. Sigma's more than 540 chapters are located at more than 700 institutions of higher education throughout Armenia, Australia, Botswana, Brazil, Canada, Chile, Colombia, Croatia, England, Eswatini, Finland, Ghana, Hong Kong, Ireland, Israel, Italy, Jamaica, Japan, Jordan, Kenya, Lebanon, Malawi, Mexico, the Netherlands, Nigeria, Pakistan, Philippines, Portugal, Puerto Rico, Scotland, Singapore, South Africa, South Korea, Sweden, Taiwan, Tanzania, Thailand, the United States, and Wales. Learn more at www.sigmanursing.org.

Sigma Theta Tau International
550 West North Street
Indianapolis, IN, USA 46202

To request a review copy for course adoption, order additional books, buy in bulk, or purchase for corporate use, contact Sigma Marketplace at 888.654.4968 (US/Canada toll-free), +1.317.687.2256 (International), or solutions@sigmamarketplace.org.

To request author information, or for speaker or other media requests, contact Sigma Marketing at 888.634.7575 (US/Canada toll-free) or +1.317.634.8171 (International).

ISBN: 9781646481606
EPUB ISBN: 9781646481613
PDF ISBN: 9781646481620

Library of Congress Control Number: 2024017420

Publisher: Dustin Sullivan

Managing Editor: Carla Hall

Acquisitions Editor: Emily Hatch

Publications Specialist: Todd Lothery

Development Editor: Rebecca Senninger

Project Editor: Rebecca Senninger

Cover Designer: Rebecca Batchelor

Copy Editor: Erin Geile

Interior Design/Page Layout: Rebecca Batchelor

Proofreader: Todd Lothery

Indexer: Larry D. Sweazy

Dedications

To Jesse, Kya, Ryelee, Julien, Evan, Killian, and Ethan.

–Jennifer

To my husband Ron, daughters Sophia and Olivia, and parents Bob and Claudia Borgna.

–Brie

Acknowledgments

We want to acknowledge all the nurses out there working every day to make staffing and scheduling better.

About the Authors

Jennifer S. Mensik Kennedy, PhD, MBA, RN, NEA-BC, FAAN, serves as the 38th president of the American Nurses Association (ANA). In this national leadership role, Mensik Kennedy boldly advocates for the nation's 5.5 million RNs. In 2023, she was named by *Modern Healthcare* as one of the 100 Most Influential People in Healthcare.

Mensik Kennedy is a sought-after presenter and prolific author based on her insights about and experience involving key nursing issues. Her books include *Lead, Drive, and Thrive in the System*, 2nd edition, and *The Nurse Manager's Guide to Innovative Staffing*, 2nd edition. She co-authored *Lead Like a Nurse*; *A Nurse's Step-By-Step Guide to Transitioning to the Professional Nurse Role*; and *The Power of Ten*, 2nd edition, and contributed a chapter to *The Career Handoff: A Healthcare Leader's Guide to Knowledge & Wisdom Transfer Across Generations*.

Prior to her presidency, Mensik Kennedy held key leadership positions within the nursing profession, including serving the American Nurses Association as Treasurer, Second Vice President, and Director-at-Large. She also served as President of the Arizona Nurses Association from 2007 to 2010. Additionally, Mensik Kennedy held the role of Governor of Nursing Practice for the Western Institute of Nursing in 2010–2014.

Mensik Kennedy earned a PhD from the University of Arizona College of Nursing with a focus on health systems and a minor in public administration from the Eller College of Management. She holds an MBA from the University of Phoenix and a BSN from Washington State University. Mensik Kennedy also earned an ADN from Wenatchee Valley College-North. Prior to assuming the presidency of ANA, she was an Associate Clinical Professor at the Oregon Health and Science University School of Nursing.

Mensik Kennedy was inducted in 2014 as a Fellow of the American Academy of Nursing. She has been recognized as Alumna of the Year by both University of Arizona College of Nursing and Washington State University College of Nursing.

She lives on her hobby farm in Oregon with her husband, Jesse, and blended family of six kids. In her free time, she enjoys gardening, camping, and traveling to see the national parks.

Brienne Sandow, MSN, RN, NEA-BC, is the Chief Operating Officer/Chief Nursing Officer (COO/CNO) of St. Luke's Meridian Medical Center and Eagle Medical Plaza, part of the St. Luke's Health System in Idaho. She has strategic oversight for both sites, working collaboratively with clinical disciplines, providers, and ancillary leaders to ensure services are fully integrated in pursuit of patient-centered outcomes. Sandow fosters a culture of partnership and commitment to high performance in all areas, focusing on exceptional staff and patient experiences, quality, safety, and efficiency of care.

In 2002, Sandow joined St. Luke's Health System. During her 21 years with the organization, she has served in multiple leadership positions and driven numerous critical initiatives. Prior to her current role, she was instrumental in supporting operations throughout the health system during the pandemic as the Director of the Enterprise Resource & Staffing Office.

Sandow earned a bachelor of science in psychology and a bachelor of science in family and consumer sciences from the University of Idaho, a bachelor of science in nursing from Boise State University, and an MSN, emphasis patient care services administration, from Sacred Heart University in Fairfield, Connecticut. She is American Nurses Credentialing Center certified in Nurse Executive Advanced.

Sandow was recently elected President of Nurse Leaders of Idaho, the local chapter of the American Organization for Nursing Leadership. She has previously served as Director-at-Large on the national ANA Board of Directors and as President of ANA Idaho. Sandow has been honored by the Women's and Children's Alliance with the Tribute to Women and Industry award and by the *Idaho Business Review* with the Accomplished Under 40 award. She is an active member of several professional organizations, including Sigma Theta Tau International Honor Society of Nursing and the American College of Healthcare Executives.

A native Idahoan, Sandow has been married to her husband Ron, a nurse practitioner, for 21 years. They have two spirited daughters: Sophia, 16, and Olivia, 12. In her free time, she enjoys relaxing by the pool, skiing, and traveling.

Additional Book Resources

To download a sample chapter and other free book resources, visit the Sigma Repository at https://sigma.nursingrepository.org/handle/10755/23769 or scan the QR code below.

Special Note to Readers

Here at Sigma, we realize that language is constantly evolving. The meaning of a word often changes over time, some words become obsolete, and some terms that were once acceptable may become controversial or even offensive, depending on the context or circumstances. We have made every effort to make language choices that are inclusive and not offensive. Should you identify words in this book that you believe negatively impact a group or groups of people, please reach out to us at Publications@SigmaNursing.org.

Table of Contents

Introduction

"The ultimate, hidden truth of the world is that it is something that we make, and could just as easily make different."
–David Graeber, *The Utopia of Rules*

Welcome to *The Nurse Manager's Guide to Innovative Staffing*! Nurse managers have one of the hardest roles in healthcare. Nurse managers often find themselves in the middle, advocating for patients, meeting the needs of their staff, all while answering to executives. Thank you for taking on this role. This is how we make change happen, stepping into discomfort and advocating for what is needed. This is especially true about staffing and scheduling.

One statement I, Jennifer, make often in interviews for TV or newspapers when asked about the nurse staffing crisis is that staffing issues didn't start with COVID-19, or after the pandemic, or because of the mass move of nurses to travel nurse positions. Staffing issues have continued for decades due to ignorance or willful non-attention to all the activities that we could do to make change happen. Managers and executives have been locked in a stalemate, arguing over what research supports or does not support, how much evidence an intervention had or did not have. Our inability, or lack of desire, to change is what got us to this point of nothing less than a staffing crisis.

As the quote from David Graeber states, every process and structure we have now was created by us. And we can change it. So as you read this book, we want you to focus on what you can change and put into practice. How is your organization and unit structured now? Does your staff have what they need today? We cannot constantly burden direct care nurses and clinicians with too much work every day and then be surprised at high turnover rates and think giving staff pizza will fix it. Nurse well-being is tied to work-life balance.

The next pandemic is not an "if" but a "when" situation. Are we ready for that? We cannot just talk about the lessons of what has happened over the last few years or decades but must actively create the system, structures, and processes so that we are always supporting the nurses who are caring for our patients.

Nurse staffing is the foundation for excellent patient care and outcomes. Decades of studies on hospital staffing and patient outcomes have given us a clear message that staffing levels impact patient outcomes. Regarding hospital staffing, what we need now is to put all this knowledge into practice and study those outcomes to find out what works or does not work related to operationalization! It is time that we, as nurses and nurse managers, do something different. Consider Albert Einstein's quote: "No problem can be solved from the same level of consciousness that created it."

Who benefits from this book? Anyone who is involved in staffing and scheduling in acute care settings. This includes charge nurses, direct care nurses, chairs of shared governance, staffing committee members, nurse managers, and other nurse leaders. Even if you are an experienced manager, we have found that many have learned so much from this book. And of course if you are new to your role, consider this part of your orientation, or the orientation for your team.

Even with decades of research on patient outcomes and nurse staffing, not much has changed in how we staff and schedule. So, the question is: How many years and decades have we thought about nurse staffing in the same way? Our profession has evolved greatly over even the last 20 years; is that reflected in how we staff to care for patients today? There is no magic bullet for solving staffing issues. It will not be found in any one method, including fixed staffing ratios or acuity-based; it can be found only in a combination of methods that takes into consideration multiple elements.

From this book, we want you to learn how to consider all aspects of the healthcare team, the meaning and profession of nursing, financials, and the many components of your unit and care delivery model, including how you organize your unit and how technology can lead to satisfied, happy nurses and excellent patient outcomes. There are so many moving parts. Your job, as a manager, is to figure out which parts work, which don't, and which ones you need. One size does not fit all in staffing.

As you tie this all together, you will need to use your resource-management and workforce-planning skills and knowledge. These are critical components as you manage and plan for your staffing and schedules. People, or your human resources, are your greatest resource and should be planned for like all other resources. In partnership with resource management, workforce planning may seem overwhelming to think about. Many times people relate workforce planning to the high-level, larger organization's or country's RN needs for the next five to 10 years, but it can be as focused as just your unit's needs for the next year. In fact, you should have an updated plan quarterly (roster management). Resource management and workforce planning are important management principles in addition to the other elements that greatly impact your staffing and scheduling.

How This Book Is Organized

Completely revised and updated, this book has three main sections.

Part I, "Understanding Staffing," gives an overview of staffing as follows:

- Chapter 1, "Nursing Fundamentals for Staffing," explores what staffing is and why it is important.

- Chapter 2, "The Current State of Staffing," reviews federal legislation; acuity-, workload-, ratio-, and budget-based methods for determining staffing; and the professional organization's role in staffing standards.

Part II addresses how to operationalize and apply research to safe staffing. There are multiple components to staffing you should think about as you go forward to determine your unit's needs. Chapters 3–8 focus on those components:

- Chapter 3, "Start With Understanding Your Unit's Care Delivery Model," reviews multiple types of care delivery models and explains why your care delivery model sets the stage for staffing.

- Chapter 4, "Maximize the Capacity and Capabilities of Your RN Workforce," addresses the role and potentially innovative practices of the RN, LPN/LVN, and nursing assistive personnel, as well as the legal scope of practice.

- Chapter 5, "Empower All Disciplines to Practice to Their Full Scope," covers the role and potential of other team members to practice and contribute to staffing and patient outcomes.

- Chapter 6, "Recognize, Manage, and Minimize Your Variability," reviews artificial and natural variability and how you can manage and eliminate issues that create havoc with your staffing and scheduling.

- Chapter 7, "Target Technology That Improves Staffing and Outcomes," considers various technology solutions and the impact on budget, staffing, and outcomes.

- Chapter 8, "Pulling Your Data Together," explains how to get your staffing and scheduling numbers as well as how to deal with scheduling issues such as holidays, vacation, and leave.

Part III, "Staffing Tools and Models," includes Chapters 9–11 and the Epilogue:

- Chapter 9, "Innovative Care Delivery Models," discusses rural and Critical Access Hospital staffing, as well as specialty unit staffing models. It also addresses emergency management and pandemic response.

- Chapter 10, "Outside the Hospital Walls," is a new chapter that addresses staffing along the care continuum in this time of healthcare reform.

- Chapter 11, "Examples of Staffing Plans, Policies, and Committees," offers great examples of documents and processes used by others in the real world.

- The Epilogue highlights some of the most important takeaways from this book.

Each chapter in this book offers practical advice, personal experiences, tips, things to consider, and examples. Many of the examples come from RNs who have experience managing a unit or department. Some of these examples are about innovative programs, and others are about things that may not have worked as well as had been hoped.

In addition to great shared experiences, the book provides examples, forms, samples, calculations, and sample processes that can inform your staffing and scheduling decisions. This book is a starting point for staffing and scheduling. For those who have been managing for a while and never had any formal education in staffing and scheduling, this book will provide you with information that you can use to orient your new managers. For those who are new or considering a management position, this book will be foundational for you as you learn to be a manager. This book provides a starting point for you.

A Shift in Thinking

Regardless of how many years someone has been a nurse, they need to put aside what they know unless it is evidence-based. Experiences are important, but alone they are not sufficient to advance their knowledge. Experiences can bias how someone thinks about something new. Now, is it possible to be completely unbiased? No. But we want you to incorporate evidence and think differently about all aspects of your staffing. Does this also mean that there is sufficient evidence out there on different care delivery models? No, there isn't. There will never be a randomized controlled trial of staffing levels, as that would be unethical. As humans, we will always make decisions within a framework of bounded rationality. We will never have all the information needed to make a decision. But decisions must be made to progress.

Let us see a change in your thinking. We want you to think about staffing in a drastically different way. Do not just think about how staffing worked or did not work when you were a staff nurse. Remember, no problem can be solved from the same level of consciousness that created it.

In the end, our hope is that you learn something that can be applied today; that you take what you learn and make a difference in your unit/your staff's work environment; and, most importantly, that you positively impact your patients. We owe safe staffing to our patients and their families. They have entrusted us with their lives and loved ones.

Nurses have been the most trusted profession for more than two decades now. Let's continue to earn that trust by bringing new and innovative thinking to our work every day.

PART 1

Understanding Staffing

Nursing Fundamentals for Staffing

All direct care RNs, at one point or another, have been subjected to the ups and downs of the department's scheduling process. You may have even wondered who created the schedule and what they were thinking when they created it. We have all had those days where we felt there were not enough staff to provide the level of care we believed our patients deserved. Many of us thought, "If we were in charge, we would do it right!" Now that you are a nurse manager, do you still feel that way? Maybe even more important, are you doing it the "right way"? What is the right way anyhow? Well, this book is your opportunity to learn how to staff and schedule the right way. You will learn methods and techniques you can apply to your department to schedule and maintain the appropriate number of personnel on a given shift to ensure the highest quality of patient care—while staying within budget. This of course assumes that patient care needs drive the budget, not the other way around. And if your organization is not savvy, the content of this book will help you get there.

In this chapter, we discuss the definition of nursing and the importance of the nursing process, and we define staffing. We also touch on patient-flow variability and how nurse staffing research has demonstrated a positive relationship between patient outcomes and staff satisfaction. From this chapter, we want you to take away quantifiable outcomes, which you can share with others, that point out the importance of staffing to high-quality and safe patient care. We also want you to understand that the fundamentals—the definition of nursing and the nursing process you learned about in your prelicensure program—are alive and well today. Staffing and scheduling to ensure the entire nursing process is completed for each and every patient, and that there is no missed care, is a fundamental essential to each and every one of our nursing licenses.

Ensuring High-Quality Patient Care

Nursing is a profession, and there are many aspects to professional nursing besides the technical or hands-on clinical interventions nurses perform (see Table 1.1). We are not saying technical tasks are unimportant, but somewhere along the line, RNs and their patients began to think that the technical side is the only role of the nurse. At one point in history, RNs could not start IVs or use a stethoscope. Is it time to rethink what RNs do and delegate some of those tasks to others? The technical tasks are the "interventions" of professional practice. RNs spend most of their time on interventions and far too little on the other components of their professional practice such as reassessment after the completed intervention. Basing your staffing solely on these quantifiable tasks would never fully capture the essence of or allow enough time per nurse per shift for much of the most important nursing work. It also results in missed care for the patient and moral distress among your staff.

TABLE 1.1   ANA STANDARDS OF PRACTICE, 2021

Professional Practice (Nursing Process)	Technical or "Task"-Based Practice (Standard 5: Implementation step as main focus in the nursing process)
Standard 1: Assessment	Administer medications and injections
Standard 2: Diagnosis	Dress wounds and incisions
Standard 3: Outcomes Identification	Perform routine laboratory work
Standard 4: Planning	Start and maintain IVs and central line dressings
Standard 5: Implementation	Assist physicians in examinations and during surgeries
	Administer IV medications
	Track and record vital signs
Standard 5A: Coordination of Care	Insert and maintain catheters
Standard 5B: Health Teaching and Health Promotion	Assist with personal hygiene and dressing
Standard 6: Evaluation	Change patient position and ambulation

Reach back into your memory and imagine yourself sitting in nursing school when you were first introduced to the nursing process. Recall those high-quality nursing care plans you feverishly worked on the night before your clinical rotations. Once you found yourself in the real nursing world, did you continue to create those nursing care plans, or did you find yourself doing only interventions, with your care plans nowhere in sight? If you were like many nurses, you realized as a new nurse, you didn't have the time to fully practice nursing like you were taught—what we consider the gold standard. You were forced to prioritize and even ration the care you could give. There was only so much time in the shift to pass medications, complete documentation, and not get in trouble for incremental overtime for staying past your shift to get care done. As time progressed, you settled into the new norm for substandard nursing care. You focused your valuable time on what you thought were the most important tasks of nursing—or the only tasks you could handle as you struggled with the workload. You allowed the system to dictate and control your nursing practice even though you are the one who holds a nursing license.

Remember these two important foundational pieces:

1. Understanding the definition of nursing

2. Understanding the process of nursing

We discuss both the definition and process of nursing in the following sections.

What Is Nursing?

This book uses the American Nurses Association (ANA) definition of *nursing:*

> Nursing integrates the art and science of caring and focuses on the protection, promotion, and optimization of health and human functioning; prevention of illness and injury; facilitation of healing; and alleviation of suffering through compassionate presence. Nursing is the diagnosis and treatment of human responses and advocacy in the care of individuals, families, groups, communities, and populations in recognition of the connection of all humanity. (ANA, 2021, p. 1)

But why use the ANA definition, you might ask? Maybe your organization has its own definition of nursing. The importance of using a standard definition of nursing is that you can more effectively communicate the outcomes of your work on staffing and patient care to finance personnel, administration, your boss, and your colleagues when everyone works from the same page. When we are on the same page, we can start to do such things as compare outcomes and request additional nursing resources because we have a collective standard platform. Also, the ANA is a professional organization representing all registered nurses.

What Is the Nursing Process?

The *nursing process* is an outcome-oriented method of nursing that provides a framework to guide care. Although many of you probably remember a five-step nursing process, the current process added several more steps, as noted in Table 1.1.

Some nursing theorists and managers feel that the nursing process is outdated and linear. We believe it is linear only if you make it that way. Whatever your belief, the nursing process gives a name to each of the steps and helps nurses step back from nursing being a task-oriented process. Nursing should be a patient-centered approach that is built upon both the ANA standards of practice and the standards of professional performance (see Table 1.2).

TABLE 1.2 ANA STANDARDS OF PRACTICE AND PROFESSIONAL PERFORMANCE (ANA, 2021)

Standards of Practice	Standards of Professional Performance
Standard 1: Assessment	Standard 7: Ethics
Standard 2: Diagnosis	Standard 8: Advocacy
Standard 3: Outcomes Identification	Standard 9: Respectful and Equitable Practice
Standard 4: Planning	Standard 10: Communication
Standard 5: Implementation	Standard 11: Collaboration
Standard 5A: Coordination of Care	Standard 12: Leadership
Standard 5B: Health Teaching and Health Promotion	Standard 13: Education
Standard 6: Evaluation	Standard 14: Scholarly Inquiry
	Standard 15: Quality of Practice
	Standard 16: Professional Practice Evaluation
	Standard 17: Resource Stewardship
	Standard 18: Environmental Health

Without the nursing process being evident in its entirety, hospital administrators and nurse managers alike will continue to staff and budget for nurses to perform only the implementation/intervention components in the nursing process. It is only in performing the *entire* nursing process, however, that nurses find satisfaction and reward in their work. Satisfied nurses are less likely to leave an organization or their manager, giving you a more experienced workforce that leads to improved patient experiences and outcomes. (Chapter 2 further dives into research around the importance of nurse satisfaction.) When nurses utilize the entire process as designed, they will spend more time at the bedside with their patients.

It is essential that all nurse managers and staff nurses understand what they can and cannot delegate when using the nursing process. All state boards of nursing have rules and regulations that specify RN scope, LPN scope, and what can be delegated to nursing assistive personnel (NAP). Many times we have heard that an LPN has "assessed or evaluated a patient," which, in many states, is beyond the scope of LPN practice. We then often hear that either the MD or RN has signed off on this assessment, as if that makes it OK. As a nurse manager, you need to understand the principles of delegation and your state board rules and regulations before you staff your unit. Since the COVID-19 pandemic, many states have added safe harbor laws that allow nurses to escalate without fear of retribution instances of unsafe care and/or practice. Do not place your nursing staff in precarious situations regarding their licenses. (See Chapter 5, which includes further discussion on state boards and scope.)

NOTE

Know the scope of practice of each member of your team. Just because staff members have always done something on your unit or in your hospital does not mean it is within their scope of practice. This contributes to normalization of deviance. Normalization of deviance is when individuals and teams drift from acceptable practice standards and adopt a new way of doing things that is not in alignment with current practice.

Based on the ANA Scope and Standards of Practice, an RN demonstrates authority, ownership, accountability, and responsibility for the appropriate delegation of nursing care. The RN may delegate elements of care but should not delegate the entirety of the nursing process itself. The decision to delegate should not be assumed from the fact that LPNs or NAPs are scheduled to work with RNs. The decision of whether to delegate is also based on the RN's judgment concerning the condition of the patient, the competence of all members of the nursing team, and the degree to which the RN will need to supervise if they delegate a task (Duffy & McCoy, 2014).

TIP

Staff so that your nurses have time to complete the entire nursing process, not just the interventions for their shift, or you will contribute to task-oriented nurses and increase the likelihood of patient harm and errors.

What Is Quality?

Now that you understand what nursing and the nursing process are, the next step is to understand what quality is. Because everyone in the healthcare industry seems to have a different definition of quality and an opinion on who should define it, we have adopted the National Academy of Medicine's (formerly the Institute of Medicine) dimensions of quality for the purposes of this book. The National Academy of Medicine (NAM) defines *quality* as "the degree to which health services for individuals and populations increase the likelihood of desired health outcomes and are consistent with current professional knowledge" (Cooperberg et al., 2009, p. 411). Some researchers have added suggested changes to the framework that incorporate the very important dimensions of quality while adding new components with equity and value cutting across all (Bau et al., 2019). This proposed updated framework provides the users the ability to focus on measuring both healthcare quality and disparities:

1. Safety

2. Timeliness

3. Efficiency

4. Effectiveness

5. Access

6. Patient/family-centeredness

7. Care coordination

8. Health systems infrastructure capabilities

As we know that nurse staffing impacts quality, consider the five guiding principles that serve as guideposts for building sustainable nurse staffing structures and models in looking at quality. These five principles are (Nurse Staffing Task Force, 2023):

1. Safe

2. Accountable

3. Transformative

4. Equitable

5. Collaborative

The NAM framework and five guideposts should always be at the forefront of your staffing decisions when creating new models of care and when determining a schedule that is nurse driven.

Understanding Staffing and Your Patient-Flow Variability

Start to think about your unit or when you practiced nursing at the bedside. Did crazy things always seem to happen during a full moon? Did you always experience an issue with insufficient staffing on the third Friday of the month? What are those crazy, seemingly irrational patterns in staffing that you notice repeatedly—or that have been passed down through your facility's folklore? Awareness of patterns is important, and you explore that further in Chapter 6, but here we focus on defining staffing for our purposes.

Definition of Staffing

Nurse managers know they want appropriate nurse staffing, and there are many variables to take into consideration regarding what is appropriate. We discuss all the variables that impact appropriate nurse staffing in later chapters; after considering the definition of nursing, the nursing process, and the definition of quality, we can define the terms *appropriate nurse staffing* and *scheduling*. And yes, there is a difference between the two. The Nurse Staffing Task Force (2023, para. 5) defines appropriate staffing as "a dynamic process that aligns the number of nurses, their workload, expertise, and resources with patient needs in order to achieve quality patient outcomes within a healthy work environment."

Definition of Scheduling

Merriam-Webster (n.d.) provides two definitions for scheduling:

1. A procedural plan that indicates the time and sequence of each operation

2. To appoint, assign, or designate for a fixed time

By incorporating the nursing process into staffing decisions, we have expanded the scope of the schedule to include non-nurses as well. Not all interventions and activities need to be done by nurses, after all. Nurses can delegate pieces of the nursing process to other licensed and unlicensed professionals, which is discussed in Chapter 3.

Patient-Flow Variability

In discussing staffing, start to think of your own department or unit—the flow that really leads to your challenges in staffing to begin with. If only all patients were the same, all staff were equal in experience, and patients only got sick between the hours of 8 a.m. and 5 p.m. Monday through Friday—and no holidays. But that is not the world we live in; we live in a world of variability. Take into consideration some of the ways patients are admitted to a hospital bed:

- Outside providers, such as physicians' offices or nursing homes
- Emergency departments (EDs)
- Surgical departments
- Facility-to-facility transfers
- Unit-to-unit transfers

If your hospital is like the majority, you staff to a mean (an average), not to the variability of your patient flow. While staffing to the mean upfront seems like the easiest way to go, in the long run, it is expensive, time-consuming, and emotionally draining because this staffing process does not take into consideration patient-flow variability. The major issue with variability is that your capacity does not change. You have the same number of beds and staff scheduled regardless of how few or how many patients are admitted without taking into consideration variation each hour or day of the week.

There are two types of patient-flow variability: artificial and natural (Litvak et al., 2010):

- *Artificial variability* is controlled by the hospital (e.g., when surgeries are scheduled).
- *Natural variability* just happens (e.g., the flow of ED patients). Natural variability is a result of things we cannot control (but we can plan for based on historical trending), such as tornados, earthquakes, mass-casualty events, or a bad flu season.

Artificial variability can be managed to better meet the needs of unit and hospital staffing. (This does not mean you should not do surgeries or admit patients, though, because this is your revenue source.) The only way to deal with patient-flow variability is to manage the patient flow and control census peaks. There are other components of variability to consider, which are described in Chapter 6.

To better consider your staffing situation, consider the following questions to answer and steps to take:

- Have you met with key physicians to discuss their admitting practices? As the nurse manager, you can help manage admissions on your unit; you are not totally powerless to admissions. Work with your admitting physicians to contact your unit first to help arrange a proper admission time before just sending a patient over to be admitted. Explain to the physician about the need to be able to identify the most appropriate bed on your unit as soon as possible as well as secure adequate staffing for that physician's patient. Based on the patient's condition, you may be able to move the admission a few hours to help facilitate your unit's flow of admissions and discharges.

- Does your organization have a centralized patient placement center? Work with this department staff to be the first to pull patients to keep your unit or department full so that your staff won't need to float.

- Do all the scheduled surgeries seem to occur during the first half of the week? This topic is a little touchier and more difficult to approach without the help and support of those in administration above you. When you have a bulk of scheduled surgeries in the first half of the week, you might not have enough room for patients coming through the ED or direct admissions on those days. You will have high bed usage and higher staffing needs, and your patient flow will slow and potentially increase length of stay. You will also underutilize your beds and staff in the second half of the week, which is wasted capacity.

- Do your physicians round in the morning or evening to discharge patients? If your physicians round on the sickest patients in the morning, say ICU first, and then end on the medical-surgical floor last, they might be creating a bottleneck. Physicians typically want to round on the sickest of patients first; however, the sickest patients are in intensive care, and they have the most resources and nurses monitoring them already. Orders are written in the morning to transfer to lower levels of care, but there are no beds downstream yet. Someone needs to discharge the medical-surgical patients first. Starting in medical-surgical units for rounds facilitates discharges and flow, freeing up resources downstream first so that patients can move more freely to the appropriate bed and staffing resources.

- Do you actively manage patient discharges and flow on your unit? This does not mean you have a discharge time like a hotel but that you facilitate discharges on your unit to make room for the constant flux of patients you will get. Working with the physician, your staff should be able to identify potential discharge dates that are not set in stone but are dates the team of care providers now has to work toward. Set goals for having patients discharged and off your unit by time blocks, such as 50% of patients who are to be discharged for the day have left your unit by 11 a.m. and 25% by 3 p.m. for a total of 75% of discharges occurring before evening.

- Does your unit wait to transfer patients before shift change or accept patients only after shift change? As staff nurses, we saw this happen, and as a manager, you suspect it may happen more than you want. The end of the shift is nearing, and the staff nurse would much rather have the ED nurse wait to give reports to the oncoming nurse. There are many more scenarios like this, but this action impedes patient flow. In addition, research shows an association between ED boarding and mortality (Boudi et al., 2020).

- Do you staff to the median or mode of your patient census? We discuss this more in Chapter 2, as you may find opportunities for staffing differently with the mode as opposed to the median or average. *Mode* is a set of numbers that occurs most often in a grouping of numbers. There may be no mode, one mode, or more than one mode.

- What are the paths patients take to be admitted or transferred to your unit? Map out for your unit the percentage of patients who typically come to you from the ED, direct admissions, surgery, and transfers from other units.

- Have you taken any steps to manage the artificial flow to your unit? Now that you know the percentage of your patients who come from each path, collaborate with those units' managers to streamline the flow of patients between your units. You will improve quality and patient satisfaction.

- Does your unit push or pull patients? Many units have patients "pushed" to them, which means someone calls your unit to ask you to take a patient. Pushing patients slows down the patient flow and creates wider variations in your census and staffing needs. Changing your unit's philosophy to "pulling" patients, where you or your charge nurses call looking for patients to admit to your unit, creates a stable census that decreases wide fluctuations in your staffing needs. If your unit is typically at 85% of capacity, it is easier to staff and maintain even staffing levels than to fluctuate in census and have fluctuations in staffing needs.

Patient flow has a major impact on your staffing needs. By determining artificial and natural variability, you can help manage and eliminate barriers that have a negative impact on your unit's staffing.

Why Is Staffing Important?

We touched on why staffing is important earlier, but there are more reasons to consider the importance of staffing, including legal accountability. As a nurse manager, you are held accountable to the ANA Code of Ethics for Nursing, whether or not you are a member, in a court of law and by your state board of nursing.

The ANA Code of Ethics states, "Because the nurse's primary commitment is to the patient, it carries the greatest weight and priority and consequently it trumps all other loyalties" (ANA, 2015a, p. 26). This does not say the "staff nurses'" primary commitment but "the nurse's"—singular. As a member of the profession and as a nurse, your primary commitment is to the patient. Your role in nursing is as a nurse manager, which gives you additional responsibilities to the organization (including its financial wellness) and your boss. But never forget your primary commitment, for which you are socially accountable at the expense of your role.

The ANA Social Policy Statement also speaks to the commitment and accountability you have as a professional nurse:

> Nurses, as members of a knowledge-based health profession and as licensed health care professionals, must answer to patients, nursing employers, the board of nursing, and the civil and criminal court system when the quality of patient care provided is compromised or when allegations of unprofessional, unethical, illegal, unacceptable or inappropriate nursing conduct, actions, or responses arise. (ANA, 2015b, p. 32)

It is important to understand your professional, societal, and organizational responsibilities to staffing. You place your staff and patients at risk, as well as yourself, when you staff with the mindset of meeting your budget or a set of staff ratios only.

NOTE

In staffing your unit, you are legally and professionally accountable and responsible to your patients, staff, organization, and society.

The Healthcare Environment

Every generation believes it is living in the most challenging of times, but for healthcare, the US is at a pivotal point on the heels of the COVID-19 pandemic. Rising salaries and hospitals attempting to quickly recapture several years of losses incurred from the COVID-19 pandemic are both causing skyrocketing healthcare costs. Most of us probably agree that we should spend less on healthcare.

We need to find innovative ways to provide quality patient care with the money that is already spent on healthcare in the US (Mensik Kennedy, 2023). The Centers for Disease Control and Prevention (CDC) notes that in 2019 the US spent $11,582 per capita on healthcare (CDC/National Center for Health

Statistics, 2022). Additionally, of the total spend, 31.4% of total expenditures were for hospital care (CDC/National Center for Health Statistics, 2022).

Of the US's total healthcare spending, it has been estimated that 25% of spending is on waste (Shrank et al., 2019). Examples of waste include failure of care delivery, failure of care coordination, and administrative complexity (Shrank et al., 2019).

A review found the following estimate ranges for the cost of waste (Shrank et al., 2019):

- Failure of care delivery: $102.4 billion to $165.7 billion
- Failure of care coordination: $27.2 billion to $78.2 billion
- Overtreatment or low-value care: $75.7 billion to $101.2 billion
- Pricing failure: $230.7 billion to $240.5 billion
- Fraud and abuse: $58.5 billion to $83.9 billion
- Administrative complexity: $265.6 billion

As well, the Commonwealth Fund recently published a report titled "High U.S. Health Care Spending: Where Is It All Going?" The report noted that reductions in administrative burdens and drug costs could substantially reduce the difference between US and peer nation health spending by up to 45% (Turner et al., 2023). While there has been an effort to address waste in numerous studies, we found no studies through 2019 focused on interventions to decrease administrative complexity (Shrank et al., 2019).

So, what does this have to do with staffing? Remember the definition of quality? It includes being efficient. It may be easier to schedule as many nurses as possible, but it is not efficient. As a nurse manager, you have the responsibility to produce quality patient care while being as efficient as possible. Keep in mind that "treating the health care system like a (wildly inefficient) jobs program conflicts directly with the goal of ensuring that all Americans have access to care at an affordable price" (Baicker & Chandra, 2012, p. 2435). An article from *The New York Times* in 1990 lamented rising healthcare costs at that time, noting that the more we spend, the less we spend on other social needs. Further, the article pointed out that CEO salaries and bond staff contributed to a significant amount of waste (Hilts, 1990). Here we are over 30+ years later and not much has changed.

Not taking significant steps to control health spending could mean job losses for other workers. There is only so much money to spend on healthcare; the more money spent on healthcare, the less money is available for other essential and non-essential goods and services. A promising step for healthcare reform can be found in value-based care, Medicare's Shared Savings Program, and Accountable Care Organizations, which are discussed later in this chapter.

Appropriate Resource Utilization and Stewardship

Resource stewardship is one of the standards of professional practice for RNs. It is the RN's responsibility to "utilize appropriate resources to plan, provide, and sustain evidence-based nursing services that are safe, effective, financially responsible, and used judiciously" (ANA, 2021, p. 105). This includes advocating for equitable resources, securing appropriate resources to address needs, and addressing discriminatory healthcare practices (ANA, 2021). This is a complex issue. In consideration of lower costs, how can appropriate nurse staffing be fiscally responsible? Can we place a dollar amount to providing care that does no harm to the individual patient?

In the argument for appropriate nurse-staffing levels, a manager can improve nurse satisfaction, which in turn decreases nurse turnover (think of costs to rehire and train) and decreases adverse patient outcomes. The Centers for Medicare & Medicaid Services (CMS) has implemented a policy of refusing to pay medical claims based on hospital-acquired conditions—and rightfully so. If you took your car to a mechanic, you would expect them to fix everything that needed to be fixed but not cause additional problems that you would need to pay for. Why should a patient pay for, or a private or government payer reimburse for, conditions hospitals could have prevented had their staffing been appropriate?

However, the responsibility to save and reduce costs should not be placed solely on the nursing profession. All too often, nursing care is seen as an expense and not as a revenue producer for a healthcare organization. Each additional patient-care RN employed (at 7.8 hours per patient day) is estimated to generate more than $60,000 annually in reduced medical costs and improved national productivity (Dall et al., 2009). Nurse managers manage this magic number. Not too many and not too few staff for your unit!

NOTE

Should managers staff more nurses or should patients have longer stays? In one study, in addition to producing better outcomes, the costs avoided due to fewer readmissions and shorter lengths of stay (LOS) were more than twice the cost of the additional nurse staffing (McHugh et al., 2021).

More Is Not Always Better: Roster Management

Have you ever considered overstaffing or overhiring just to make sure you have the staff to take care of the patients when you need them? At first glance, that may seem like a potential solution to your staffing issues, but in the long run, it can have devastating effects. While being above budget on labor costs, you might be managing overtime and mandatory low census week to week. This is where roster management comes in handy, which may still be called *position control* in some organizations.

The difference between position control and roster management is that in position control, staff are hired, managed, and leveraged based on volume; in roster management, staff are organized and allocated to meet business needs and demands. Roster management aims to ensure adequate staff coverage at all times while considering the competencies and skills of each nurse. If your organization has roster management, ask about it and understand how it impacts you. If your organization does not have a roster management process or is focused mainly on a position control philosophy, you can implement one for your unit. (Roster management is discussed further in Chapter 8.)

Research

A lot of useful information comes from research on nurse staffing, much of which can be used as support when arguing the need to increase staffing, increase a full-time equivalent, or explain your budget variance. Research has demonstrated the impact of staffing on nurse satisfaction and patient outcomes (Lake et al., 2019): The lower the staffing, the lower the staff satisfaction. Also, the lower the staffing, the worse outcomes are, particularly nursing-sensitive outcomes.

The Missing Component: Missed Care

Missed care has been studied for well over a decade, but more recently this topic has been brought to life. *Missed care* is any aspect of required patient care that is omitted or delayed (Kalisch et al., 2009). Missed care occurs by omission and commission. Missed care by commission is believed to be the most common but often is unreported. Examples of missed care include:

- Communication and information sharing (Bagnasco et al., 2020)

- Self-management, autonomy, and education including care planning, discharge planning, and decision-making (Bagnasco et al., 2020)

- Fundamental physical care (Bagnasco et al., 2020)

- Emotional and psychological care including spiritual care (Bagnasco et al., 2020)

- Nurse-initiated independent interventions (Mandal et al., 2020)

- Patient surveillance (Mandal et al., 2020)

- Medication administration (Mandal et al., 2020)

- Symptom management (Mandal et al., 2020)

Missed nursing care is often the result of poor staffing, not just inappropriate resource management. When faced with not enough staff or time, decisions to ration and prioritize care are made based on what is the most immediate need. Missed and rationed care contributes to moral distress and higher burnout levels in nurses (Abdelhadi et al., 2022). (As will be discussed throughout this book, there are clear connections between staffing levels and outcomes.)

The Impact of Staffing on Patients

What other impact does staffing have on patient outcomes? As pressure increases in the drive to decrease healthcare costs, nurses have already demonstrated the impact of staffing on patient outcomes through research and the use of nursing-sensitive indicators. Nursing-sensitive indicators include:

- Catheter-associated urinary tract infections
- Falls
- Pressure ulcers
- Intravenous infiltrations
- Nosocomial infections
- Restraint usage
- Pain management
- Pneumonia
- Shock
- Upper gastrointestinal bleeding
- Longer length of hospital stays
- Failure to rescue
- 30-day mortality

The Agency for Healthcare Research and Quality (Stanton, 2004) funded multiple studies focusing on nurse staffing and outcomes and published those findings more than a decade ago. There should be no doubt that nurse staffing impacts patient outcomes. Additionally, research shows that better nurse staffing does impact other patient outcomes such as decreases in mortality (all causes), decreases in mortality inpatient, decreased healthcare-associated infections, reduced hazard of experiencing adverse events, and decreased length of stay among others (Dall'Ora et al., 2023). The most quoted statistic is from Linda Aiken and Associates, where they found each additional patient per nurse was associated with a 7% increase in the likelihood of dying within 30 days of admission and a 7% increase in the odds of failure to rescue (Aiken et al., 2013).

These results are just a few of the many outcomes discovered through research. You probably have personal stories about how staffing may or may not have had positive impacts on patient outcomes. Regardless of your type of unit, you have many opportunities to quantify and demonstrate the relationship between your unit's quality measures. Some measures may be collected as mandatory and others as voluntary. Your organization may use different vendors for collection. Some of the quality data collected may be repetitive.

Manager Exercise

Think about the ways you or your nurses have experienced the impact of nurse staffing on patient outcomes. Write them down. You need to ensure you communicate your unit's patient outcomes, both positive and negative, to support your nurse-staffing needs. What is your pressure ulcer rate? Have you positively impacted patient falls? Have you correlated your nursing-sensitive indicators to your staffing levels?

TIP

If you do not have access to your unit's quality data in a timely manner, ask for it. It is hard to make changes in patient outcomes and staffing with data that is three months old.

Your organization can collect multiple pieces of data that are important for you to know and review. To compare your staffing with patient outcomes, you can use data from the following sources:

- National Patient Safety Goals (Joint Commission): http://www. jointcommission.org/standards/national-patient-safety-goals/

- National Database for Nursing Quality Indicators: https://www.pressganey.com/platform/ndnqi

- CMS Core Measures: https://www.cms.gov/medicare/quality/measures/ core-measures

- Leapfrog Group: http://leapfroggroup.org

- State-specific requirements

It is important to note that information from any one organization can change or be updated at any given time. Always make sure that you refer to these organizations' websites for the most up-to-date information. This is not an exhaustive list; however, it is one that will get you started in the right direction. If your hospital takes Medicare patients, you will have CMS core measure data. However, if you are a Critical Access Hospital or a hospital with fewer than 25 licensed acute care beds, your hospital is exempt from collecting or reporting certain data points. Based on the size of your unit or the size of your hospital, your sample size for outcome data may be small, inconsistent, or nonexistent month to month, making it hard to use as a data-analysis point to understand the effectiveness of your staffing.

How Much Data Do You Need?

For a small organization or unit, use the average, or mean, of both quality and staffing data over a quarter or a year to have a meaningful analysis. For a larger unit or organization, it may be possible to use monthly or weekly data to make a meaningful analysis between patient outcomes and staffing.

The Impact of Staffing on Staff

The original Magnet® hospital work came during the nursing shortage in the early 1980s. During that time, it was noted that some hospitals in the same town may have experienced a shortage, whereas others had more candidates for positions than they could hire. Based on research and further understanding of why those hospitals may not have experienced the effects of a nursing shortage, those units were dubbed *Magnet hospitals* for their ability to attract and retain nurses. To understand this issue, the Governing Council of the American Academy of Nursing appointed the Task Force on Nursing Practice in Hospitals in 1981, charging it to examine characteristics of systems that foster or impede professional nursing practice in hospitals (McClure & Hinshaw, 2002). The study, "Magnet Hospitals: Attraction and Retention of Professional Nurses," was the impetus for understanding why not every hospital experienced a nursing shortage. Specific findings of the study included the following:

- Quality of staff was apparently viewed to be as important as quantity.

- Magnet hospitals did not employ nurses from temporary agencies.

- Magnet hospitals employed clinical specialists who were seen as valuable resources to staff as well as enriching the practice environment.

- Shift rotation was minimized, if not eliminated.

- Great efforts were made to reduce the number of weekends that nurses were required to work.

- A number of creative and flexible arrangements had been developed that were tailored to meet the needs of the personal lives of staff.

These findings, while more than 40 years old, are still relevant. Since that time, researchers have continued to study nurse satisfaction and refine and update this original study. Findings continue to show that satisfied nurses are less likely to leave an organization (Aiken et al., 2002; Kramer & Schmalenberg, 2008; Kutney-Lee et al., 2015). Although nurse satisfaction has several components, the focus throughout this book is on staffing. You will not have trouble finding nurses for your unit if they believe they will have sufficient staffing to provide quality patient care. Not only will you have plenty of staff to schedule—your unit costs will be less because you will have lower turnover and orientation costs.

> **NOTE**
>
> *The average cost of turnover for a staff RN is $52,350, with the range averaging from $40,200 to $64,500. However, less than half of hospitals collect this data (NSI Nursing Solutions, 2023).*

Value-Based Care

Medicare Shared Savings, Accountable Care Organizations (ACOs), and value-based care are relatively newer terms that often are used, sometimes inappropriately, when discussing healthcare reform. If you don't have day-to-day experience with these, they can be confusing, and you may be tempted to brush it aside when it comes to nurse staffing. As payment reform continues, albeit slowly, healthcare organizations are trying to be proactive within a value-based care framework in anticipation of future revenue impact.

The *Medicare Shared Savings Program* (MSSP) is a voluntary program that encourages groups of providers, hospitals, and other healthcare providers to come together with an ACO to provide high-quality care. The MSSP provides clarity and a certain protection when organizations and independent providers work together to provide certain contracted care that otherwise might be deemed unlawful under antitrust laws. MSSP facilitates coordination and cooperation among providers to improve the quality of care for Medicare fee-for-service (FFS) beneficiaries and reduce unnecessary costs (see Figure 1.1). Eligible providers, hospitals, and suppliers may participate in the MSSP by creating or participating in an ACO (CMS, n.d.). MSSP is designed to improve beneficiary outcomes and increase value of care by:

- Promoting accountability for a patient population

- Coordinating items and services for Medicare FFS beneficiaries

- Encouraging investment in high-quality and efficient services

Current Method of Billing Services

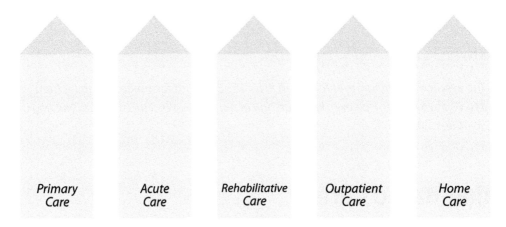

Primary Care Acute Care Rehabilitative Care Outpatient Care Home Care

Each Type of Service Bills Independent of the Other Services

FIGURE 1.1

The current reimbursement model.

Value-based care is designed to focus on quality, provider performance, and the patient experience (CMS, n.d.). The CMS definition of an ACO is a "group of doctors, hospitals, and other healthcare providers, who come together voluntarily to give coordinated high-quality care to their Medicare patients" (CMS, n.d., para. 1). An ACO can include—but is not limited to—clinics, hospitals, insurance payers, home health agencies, dialysis centers, and nursing homes.

Although participation in an ACO is purely voluntary, many organizations have seen the potential benefit and understand that they need to change—not only to be successful but also because it is the right thing to do. Doesn't this make sense—healthcare organizations partnering and working together? The program is designed to allow these partnerships to exist without violating federal laws—such as anti-trust, anti-kickback, and physician self-referral—that govern appropriate competition in the healthcare marketplace.

Payment Structure Example for a CHF Patient in an ACO Model
Mary M. is an 84-year-old congestive heart failure (CHF) patient with Medicare FFS as her insurance. Her provider and local community hospital have decided to participate in MSSP as part of an ACO. Mary saw her physician for exacerbation of her CHF symptoms; however, two days later she was admitted to the local hospital. After her discharge from the hospital, Mary was seen by the home care agency to assist in managing her symptoms. The ACO will get a bundled payment for this "episode" from CMS and has already determined through prior agreements which organization gets paid and how much they will get paid for the care provided. Thus, they are more accountable together for providing cost-effective, quality care.

Because acute care hospitalizations consume a majority of healthcare dollars, an ACO needs to reduce hospital admissions, not just readmissions, to reduce healthcare spending. More nurses will be needed outside hospital walls to coordinate care among all these providers, and fewer nurses will be needed to provide acute care in hospitals.

In the last decade, ACOs have saved Medicare over $21 billion in gross savings and $1.8 billion in 2022 alone (CMS, n.d.). As of 2023, there are 483 Medicare ACOs serving 11 million Medicare beneficiaries. Since 2010, over 1,200 organizations have held ACO contracts. Your staffing decisions will be impacted if your organization moves toward an ACO model of care. Becoming an ACO may impact your unit in the following ways:

- Shorter lengths of stay

- Increased use of post-acute services

- Increased transparency of your quality measures to other organizations in the ACO

- Shared reimbursement for a patient, potentially resulting in less reimbursement for acute care services than received today

- Redesign of care delivery on your unit

Healthcare reform is moving healthcare organizations to do a better job of care coordination, which will increase quality patient care while reducing costs. New models of care delivery under ACOs will continue to develop that will have major implications for nurse staffing now and in the future.

Summary

Here are the key points covered in this chapter:

- Quality care is safe, equitable, efficient, effective, timely, and patient-centered.

- Per the ANA Code of Ethics and social policy statement, you have an ethical responsibility to ensure nurse staffing that delivers quality patient care.

- How you staff your unit may contribute to either task-oriented nurses or RNs working at the top of their license, so use the entire nursing process as you develop staff guidelines.

- Research has demonstrated that nurse staffing impacts the quality and safety of patient care as well as nurse satisfaction.

- Understanding your unit's natural and artificial variability in patient flow enables you to manage it, not become a victim of it.

References

Abdelhadi, N., Drach-Zahavy, A., & Srulovici, E. (2022). Work interruptions and missed nursing care: A necessary evil or an opportunity? The role of nurses' sense of controllability. *Nursing Open, 9*(1), 309–319. https://doi.org/10.1002/nop2.1064

Aiken, L. H., Clarke, S. P., Sloane, D. M., Sochalski, J. A., & Silber, J. H. (2002). Hospital nurse staffing and patient mortality, nurse burnout, and job dissatisfaction. *Journal of the American Medical Association, 288*(16), 1987–1993. https://doi.org/10.1001/jama.288.16.1987

Aiken, L. H., Sloane, D. M., Bruyneel, L., Van den Heede, K., & Sermeus, W. (2013). Nurses' reports of working conditions and hospital quality of care in 12 countries in Europe. *International Journal of Nursing Studies, 50*, 43–153. https://doi.org/10.1016/j.ijnurstu.2012.11.009

American Nurses Association. (2015a). *Code of ethics for nurses with interpretive statements: Development, interpretation, and application* (2nd edition). Author.

American Nurses Association. (2015b). *Nursing's social policy statement* (2nd ed.). Author.

American Nurses Association. (2021). *Nursing: Scope and standards of practice* (4th ed.). Author.

Bagnasco, A., Dasso, N., Rossi, S., Galanti, C., Varone, G., Catania, G., Zanini, M., Aleo, G., Watson, R., Hayter, M., & Sasso, L. (2020). Unmet nursing care needs on medical and surgical wards: A scoping review of patients' perspectives. *Journal of Clinical Nursing, 29*(3–4), 347–369. https://doi.org/10.1111/jocn.15089

Baicker, K., & Chandra, A. (2012). The health care jobs fallacy. *The New England Journal of Medicine, (366)*26, 2433–2435.

Bau, I., Logan, R. A., Dezii, C., Rosof, B., Fernandez, A., Paasche-Orlow, M. K., & Wong, W. F. (2019). Patient-centered, integrated health care quality measures could improve health literacy, language access, and cultural competence. *NAM Perspectives.* Discussion paper, National Academy of Medicine. https://doi.org/10.31478/201902a

Boudi, Z., Lauque, D., Alsabri, M., Östlundh, L., Oneyji, C., Khalemsky, A., Rial, C. L., Liu, S. W., Camargo Jr., C. A., Aburawi, E., Moeckel, M., Slagman, A., Christ, M., Singer, A., Tazarourte, K., Rathlev, N. K., Grossman, S. A., & Bellou, A. (2020). Association between boarding in the emergency department and in-hospital mortality: A systematic review. *PLoS One, 15*(4), e0231253. https://doi.org/10.1371/journal.pone.0231253

Centers for Disease Control, National Center for Health Statistics. (2022). *Health expenditures.* https://www.cdc.gov/nchs/fastats/health-expenditures.htm

Centers for Medicare & Medicaid Services. (n.d.). *Accountable Care Organizations (ACOs): General information.* https://innovation.cms.gov/innovation-models/aco

Cooperberg, M. R., Birkmeyer, J. D., & Litwin, M. S. (2009). Defining high quality health care. In *Urologiconcology: Seminars and original investigations, (27)*4, 411–416. Elsevier.

Dall, T. M., Chen, Y. J., Seifert, R. F., Maddox, P. J., & Hogan, P. F. (2009). The economic value of professional nursing. *Medical Care, 47*(1), 97–104. https://doi.org/10.1097/MLR.0b013e3181844da8

Dall'Ora, C., Ejebu, O.-Z., Ball, J., & Griffiths, P. (2023). Shift work characteristics and burnout among nurses: Cross-sectional survey. *Occupational Medicine, 73*(4), 199–204. https://doi.org/10.1093/occmed/kqad046

Duffy, M., & McCoy, S. F. (2014). *Delegation and YOU!* Nursing World.

Hilts, P. (1990, Nov. 1). U.S. health care costs soar, but not as much in New York. *The New York Times.* https://www.nytimes.com/1990/11/01/us/us-health-care-costs-soar-but-not-as-much-in-new-york.html

Kalisch, B. J., Landstrom, G., & Williams, R. A. (2009). Missed nursing care: Errors of omission. *Nursing Outlook, 57*(1), 3–9. https://doi.org/10.1016/j.outlook.2008.05.007

Kramer, M., & Schmalenberg, C. (2008). Confirmation of a healthy work environment. *Critical Care Nurse, 28*(2), 56–63.

Kutney-Lee, A., Stimpfel, A. W., Sloane, D. M., Cimiotti, J. P., Quinn, L. W., & Aiken, L. H. (2015). Changes in patient and nurse outcomes associated with Magnet hospital recognition. *Medical Care, 53*(6), 550–557. https://doi.org/10.1097/MLR.0000000000000355

Lake, E. T., Sanders, J., Duan, R., Riman, K. A., Schoenauer, K. M., & Chen, Y. (2019). A meta-analysis of the associations between the nurse work environment in hospitals and 4 sets of outcomes. *Medical Care, 57*(5), 353–361. https://doi.org/10.1097/MLR.0000000000001109

Litvak, E., Vaswani, S. G., Long, M. C., & Prenney, B. (2010). Managing variability in healthcare delivery. In *The healthcare imperative: Lowering costs and improving outcomes: Institute of Medicine workshop summary* (pp. 294–301). The National Academies Press.

Mandal, L., Seethalakshmi, A., & Rajendrababu, A. (2020). Rationing of nursing care, a deviation from holistic nursing: A systematic review. *Nursing Philosophy, 21*(1), e12257. https://doi.org/10.1111/nup.12257

McClure, M. L., & Hinshaw, A. S. (Eds.). (2002). *Magnet hospitals revisited: Attraction and retention of professional nurses.* American Nurses Association.

McHugh, M. D., Aiken, L. H., Sloane, D. M., Windsor, C. D., & Yates, P. (2021). Effects of nurse-to-patient ratio legislation on nurse staffing and patient mortality, readmissions, and length of stay: A prospective study in a panel of hospitals. *Lancet, 397*(10288), 1905–1913. https://doi.org/10.1016/S0140-6736(21)00768-6

Mensik Kennedy, J. (2023). *Lead, drive, and thrive in the system* (2nd ed.). American Nurses Association.

Merriam-Webster. (n.d.). Scheduling. In *Merriam-Webster.com dictionary.* https://www.merriam-webster.com/dictionary/scheduling

NSI Nursing Solutions. (2023). *2023 NSI national health care retention & RN staffing report.* https://www.nsinursingsolutions.com/Documents/Library/NSI_National_Health_Care_Retention_Report.pdf

Nurse Staffing Task Force. (2023). *Shaping the future of nurse staffing amidst the healthcare staffing shortage.* American Nurses Association. https://www.nursingworld.org/practice-policy/nurse-staffing/nurse-staffing-task-force

Shrank, W. H., Rogstad, T. L., & Parekh, N. (2019). Waste in the US health care system: Estimated costs and potential for savings. *Journal of the American Medical Association, 322*(15), 1501–1509. https://doi.org/10.1001/jama.2019.13978

Stanton, M. W. (2004). Hospital nurse staffing and quality of care. Agency for Healthcare Research and Quality. *Research in Action,* 14. https://www.healthwatchusa.org/downloads/nursestaffing-DHHS-2004.pdf

Turner, A., Miller, G., & Lowry, E. (2023, Oct. 4). *High U.S. health care spending: Where is it all going?* The Commonwealth Fund. https://www.commonwealthfund.org/publications/issue-briefs/2023/oct/high-us-health-care-spending-where-is-it-all-going

The Current State of Staffing

As mentioned in Chapter 1, we want quality patient care as the result of our staffing. Scheduling and staffing are complex, dynamic processes that can consume your job and take time away from other important functions such as staff interaction and patient rounds. Understanding the basics of staffing and scheduling will create a foundation of knowledge for you to build upon, one that will help keep these processes from taking over your work life. The foundation for scheduling and staffing includes understanding professional organization standards; adhering to federal and state regulations; and applying acuity-, ratio-, or finance-based methods for determining your structure. This chapter discusses professional organization standards for staffing, federal and state legislation, software programs for staffing and scheduling, and various methodologies for staffing.

The Basis for Scheduling

The schedule is not just a blank slate of holes to fill. It needs some basic information so that you have a template to start from. The basis for the schedule begins with the rules you apply to it. You start with the premise that you provide care 24 hours a day, seven days a week. This means you need to know:

- Number of staff needed for each shift

- Length of shifts

- Staffing mix for each shift (number of RNs, LPNs, and nursing assistive personnel [NAPs])

- Skill sets and competencies needed for patient care

- Unit and organization care delivery and/or staffing model

This information comes from several sources. Using only one method to determine staffing will not meet the needs of your patients; you may need to take into consideration a mix of ratio-based, workload intensity, finance-based, and/or acuity-based systems. It is important that you understand the methods behind ratio-, finance-, and acuity-based staffing methods so that you can use them to meet the needs of your patients, staff, and organization. Layered across all those methods are staffing committees. More about that a little later in this chapter.

Guide to Staffing

Many of us belong to multiple professional organizations that may have a statement or guide to staffing in a nursing specialty area. In addition, many states have some form of staffing legislation that may legislate ratios for all units or ICUs only, staffing committees, and/or public reporting.

Professional Organizations Standards

As more research is completed and more is known about staffing and outcomes, professional organization standards have changed. For instance, the Association of Women's Health, Obstetric and Neonatal Nurses (AWHONN) maintained its staffing guidelines since 2010 to take into consideration the increase in acuity and workload of nurses in this population (AWHONN, 2021). Increased nursing hours were suggested due to an increased number of women who have complications or are undergoing medical and surgical procedures, along with new technologies and documentation requirements. It is important to know what your administrators say about staffing because they may have compiled the research and made recommendations that you should take into consideration.

In Chapter 1, we define staffing and review elements of staffing based on the work of the American Nurses Association (ANA). Although the ANA does not have specific unit-level staffing guidelines, multiple specialty organizations have published guidelines. The following organizations have published staffing guidelines or position papers on staffing:

- Academy of Medical-Surgical Nurses (AMSN): www.amsn.org

- American Association of Critical-Care Nurses (AACN): www.aacn.org

- American Nurses Association (ANA): www.nursingworld.org

- Association of periOperative Registered Nurses (AORN): www.aorn.org

- Association of Women's Health, Obstetric and Neonatal Nurses (AWHONN): www.awhonn.org

- Emergency Nurses Association (ENA): www.ena.org

This list includes nursing organizations mainly by service type. There are many other nursing organizations based on population that may have position papers or suggested guidelines for staffing. It is important to review all sources of data to make evidence-based decisions.

NOTE

A professional organization's standards may be different from your state's staffing laws. Although you might want to defer to the better standard, remember you are legally bound to uphold the state's staffing legislation first.

Federal and State Regulations

The argument for improved nurse staffing has led to federal and regulatory language about staffing, in addition to a variety of enacted legislation in many states. Failure to comply with federal, regulatory, and state requirements can lead to penalties for you and your organization. It is important for you to search your local state laws to determine your state's requirements and whether you are following the intent of the law. The ANA provides some high-level information for current state legislation and regulation at nursingworld.org/practice-policy/nurse-staffing/nurse-staffing-advocacy. Additionally, you can email your state nurses association affiliated with the ANA for specifics.

For instance, federal law does not require lunch or coffee breaks, but many states have their own laws that govern this and are vastly different across different states. Do not assume that you and your facility members are complying with the law or that someone will monitor this for you. Frequently, managers find out they are in violation only after an employee, patient, or concerned family member files a complaint.

As an example, in many states, such as Oregon, violation of safe staffing regulations or not providing meal and rest breaks includes civil penalties if there is reasonable belief that safe patient care has been or may be negatively impacted. Financial penalties may be assessed up to $5,000 for no written staffing plan in place, violation of the written staffing plan, no nurse on the staffing committee, and/or hospital management not making a reasonable effort to get a replacement nurse (Department of Human Services, 2023). Additionally, civil penalties are up to $1,000 against employers for each violation of missed meals and breaks.

The following sections describe some of this legislation.

Federal Legislation

The Centers for Medicare & Medicaid Services (CMS) states in 42 Code of Federal Regulations (42CFR 482.23(b)) that it requires hospitals certified to participate in Medicare to "have adequate numbers of licensed registered nurses, licensed practical (vocational) nurses, and other personnel to provide nursing care to all patients as needed" (CMS, 2010, p. 16). Even though this regulation addresses staffing, it leads to a wide range of interpretations.

If you work at a hospital that has "deemed status," you might be surveyed not by CMS but by a different accrediting body for CMS. *Deemed status* is conferred on a hospital by an accreditation organization (e.g., The Joint Commission or DNV—Det Norske Veritas), which is formal recognition that the organization's review, continued-stay review, and medical care evaluation programs meet certain effectiveness criteria of the accreditation organization and the CMS. Being accredited by one of these organizations means that you not only have passed that organization's survey requirements but also have met CMS's standards.

The Joint Commission has stated that *staffing effectiveness* is the appropriate level of nurse staffing that will provide for the best possible outcome of individual patients throughout a particular facility. However, this has led to continued confusion on what this means and how to operationalize it. In the early 2000s, this required hospital administrators to track two human-resource indicators and two patient-outcome indicators, track data, and determine the variation in performance caused by the number, skill mix, or competency of staff. However, in June 2009, The Joint Commission suspended these standards. There was debate regarding whether there was sufficient evidence between nurse staffing and patient outcomes.

The staffing effectiveness standards of The Joint Commission became effective July 1, 2010, and will remain in effect as The Joint Commission continues to research the issues of staffing effectiveness. However, as of 2023, The Joint Commission is reconsidering this work. The current requirement states that at least once a year, the administration of a hospital/organization must provide written reports on all system or process failures, the number and type of *sentinel events* (a patient safety event that results in death, permanent harm, or severe temporary harm), information provided to families/patients about the events, and actions taken to improve patient safety. There is a separate standard for emergency staffing plans; DNV does not have patient safety goals or additional standards by which they evaluate organizations. DNV adheres to the CMS regulations as written and verifies compliance through a continuous quality-improvement lens.

Like the CMS regulation, this can still lead to various interpretations on how to operationalize across hospitals.

Up until now, CMS as a regulatory agency has stated it did not have authority to mandate minimum staffing standards. However, in 2023, CMS did submit proposed rules for minimum staffing standards in long-term care facilities. In the spring of 2024, CMS finalized this rule after reviewing public comment and has mandated minimum staffing levels in longer term care. CMS taking on this authority could also lead to stronger or clearer language related to nurse staffing in acute care hospitals.

Consider This

If you have a scope-of-service document for your unit or organization, make sure that any changes to staffing or your care delivery model are updated. Many times, individuals update only before an accrediting or regulatory body arrives. You will be held accountable for what this document states compared to what is occurring on your unit.

Congress, nursing organizations, and unions have attempted to pass federal legislation on safe staffing. Proposed federal legislation has been modeled after the California Ratios Law and has been worded to incorporate a mix of methods, including ratio- and acuity-based staffing with staff involvement. To date, no federal legislation has been passed. There have, however, been several states that have enacted some sort of legislation around staffing. Oregon became the second state in 2023 to legislate mandated staffing ratios (Washington State Nurses Association [WSNA], 2023).

State Legislation

As issues surrounding safe staffing continue, 19 states introduced some form of nurse staffing legislation in 2023. According to the ANA (2023), as of March 2022, 16 states have addressed nurse staffing either in legislation or rules. These states have enacted legislation around staffing as of 2023. Updated lists can be found at nursingworld.org (search for "staffing").

California is the only state that stipulates in law and regulations that a required minimum nurse-to-patient ratio must be maintained at all times by a unit as of 2023 (California Department of Public Health, 2008). Oregon has recently passed mandated staffing ratios as well, which includes nursing assistant minimum ratios to be implemented in 2024 (WSNA, 2023). Despite these laws, hospital administration, nurse managers, and nurses still have to wrestle with tough issues related to any staffing law or regulation. None of these laws or regulations prevent patients from coming into the emergency department (ED), and federal laws, such as the Emergency Medical Treatment and Active Labor Act, require hospitals to provide a medical screening for patients who present to the ED. Patients who may need to be admitted may continue to come to the ED, but they will stay in the ED because ratios prevent further admissions on the units if additional staff are unavailable.

Overtime is also an issue due to increased nurse fatigue, working longer than 12 hours, and decreased job and patient satisfaction (Dall'Ora et al., 2023; Stimpfel et al., 2012). There are at least 18 states with known restrictions on the use of mandatory overtime (Skinner, n.d.).

Goals for Scheduling

The number one goal of scheduling is to make sure there are enough staff available to care for your patients. To do this, we need to remember that there is a difference in the methodologies between staffing and scheduling. Managers convolute the terms staffing and scheduling all the time, and really, they are two totally separate things. Each requires different education, skills, tools, and training.

Staffing is about having the right number of adequately trained and educated people at any given time for your patients. *Scheduling* means you have the right people showing up at the right time. Not enough nurses and you are short-staffed; too many nurses and you may need to lower census staff or go over budget. If you have issues with staffing and scheduling, the results are the same: fatigue, errors, missed care, poor morale, increased turnover, and decreased satisfaction (Rerkjirattikal et al., 2020). The methods listed next will not be successful unless there is a focus on both staffing and scheduling for each.

Staffing Committees

Staffing committees are nurse-led groups that create unit- or organization-wide staffing plans based on patients' acuity and needs. State legislation may require some organizations to do this, but even if it is not required, staffing plans and/or committees are a good way to provide a collaborative approach to staffing while allowing the direct care nurse to advocate for their patients and themselves. Typically, staffing committees are majority direct care staff, such as 51% minimum, to have a greater influence in the decision-making and outcomes of the committee. These committees can create a staffing plan that matches nurse criteria with patient criteria for each shift on each type of unit. (More is discussed with examples in Chapter 11.) Four methods related to staff and scheduling are discussed here: acuity-based, workload intensity, ratio-based, and finance-based. Staffing committees can be used in conjunction with all the methods mentioned next and can use these methods with their respective data to determine the best care models.

Acuity-Based Method

The *acuity-based method* of staffing generally references the patient and is measured by the severity of disease. The acuity-based method requires using clinical judgment and considering patient characteristics. Patients are not all the same; they have varying severity of the same diagnosis, different socioeconomic statuses, and different expectations. So why do we treat staffing our units as if patients were the same? Because it is easier and because most of us lack the tools or ability to start to drill down on the differences.

This is where the usefulness of the electronic health record (EHR), nursing documentation, and the nursing process really becomes clear to staff. How many times have you heard RNs (or yourself) say that they do not understand why they have to document so much or why they have to use a care plan? Rightfully so, it seems we place data in a system only to protect us from a lawsuit. Research has noted that if health information technology is not compatible with existing workflows, it is not likely to be adopted (Moore et al., 2020). But what if the data that nurses document was used to make decisions about staffing? If you improve the perception of the impact of documentation by linking staffing the next shift to the current nursing documentation, you can be assured you will have real-time and thorough documentation. This makes your informatics nurses and staff a vital part of your staffing committees as you dive into developing your acuity standards.

Whether you use a software program or pen and paper, clinical judgment and patient characteristics are two important components to consider when staffing your unit. Here is how you use the nursing process to assist in quantifying acuity (ANA, 2021):

- **Standard 1: Assessment.** RN looks at all patient characteristics.

- **Standard 2: Diagnosis.** How many nursing-related issues need to be addressed?

- **Standard 3: Outcomes Identification.** What are the nursing-specific patient outcomes?

- **Standard 4: Planning.** This is time the nurse needs to complete various patient goals during the patient's stay.

- **Standard 5: Implementation.** This is time the nurse will spend to complete interventions or supervise those who do interventions—for example, the LPN.

- **Standard 6: Evaluation.** RN evaluates plan and makes changes as needed.

Patient characteristics may include:

- Age

- Socioeconomic status

- Family or caregivers

- Diagnosis

- Severity of illness

- Comorbidities

- Ability to provide self-care

- Length of stay

The acuity-based method of staffing is a complex process that requires you and your staff to assign a level of acuity to your patients as well as the work of the nurse. This should be work of a unit-based staffing committee. The more objective the measure, the better your "inter-rater reliability" will be among your nurses. In other words, two different nurses would be able to assess and determine the same acuity number or ranking for a patient. This method has its advantages; however, few organizations have implemented a true acuity-based model. While acuity-based staffing takes into consideration the uniqueness of each patient and their specific nursing care needs, it does require continuous review and potential updates for changes in practice and may not take into consideration workload intensity.

Workload Intensity Method

Sometimes acuity and workload intensity are used as if they are interchangeable. However, there is a difference. *Workload intensity* focuses on the amount of time that an RN spends doing different tasks. Over time, acuity doesn't always equal intensity. The workload intensity method has attempted to quantify the amount of time that it takes for all patient needs, including social, emotional, and cognitive, and then the specific care tasks might be broken down even further. So you might say in terms of how long is it taking to do medication management and the physical assessment for a behavioral health patient: The acuity of this type of patient may be low, but the intensity is high.

As an example, you could have a patient in the ICU who is sedated and could be taking less time than a behavioral health admit with a low-acuity disease but significant behavioral health needs. As more patients need behavioral health services, and there continues to be fewer services available, acute care hospitals will continue to treat and manage behavioral health patients who may not have a medical necessity for an admission. If we took into account acuity only, we may inappropriately assign not enough nurse time to this patient. Additionally, you can overlay experience and new graduate nurses with different workload intensity. A new graduate nurse just off of orientation could have a lower workload intensity of 75%, whereas an experienced nurse may have 100%.

One of the keys with intensity is that nurses have to be documenting in real time for the intensity of that patient care to be accurate. Programs that can help quantify workload intensity rely on documentation, including provider and nursing orders. This can impact workload intensity significantly, as we have all experiences where the patient's condition deteriorates and the nurse workload spikes. Once the patient condition has changed, the physician enters a set of new orders. In many programs, the nurse doesn't have to wait until all those tasks are completed and documented for them to be contributing to the workload intensity. Some programs quantify the orders and update the intensity of that patient once the orders are entered. The benefit is that you can make appropriate assignments for nurses or update assignments throughout the day, especially in light of any admissions or patients transferring in. You may not give that nurse another patient based on an updated view of their workload intensity.

Ratio-Based Method

Ratio-based staffing may be the easiest method. If you plan to have a ratio of 1:5 on a medical-surgical floor, then you ensure you have one nurse for every five patients. Based on this number, it is easy to flex your staffing up and down based solely on the number of patients you have. Arguments for ratios state, "You have to start somewhere." This is true. There is always a minimum number of nurses needed to staff a unit. Staff and managers alike refer to this as their *staffing ratio*. Staffing by ratios does not come only from mandated legislation. Often this ratio is derived from the finance-based method, where nurse managers are given an hour per patient day target from the finance department. This then gets translated into a specific number of nurses, and in turn, that specific number of nurses split the patients on the unit, thus a ratio.

Staff and managers should not settle for pure ratio staffing. There should be an understanding that other factors need to be taken into consideration, such as the following:

- Patient acuity

- Workload intensity

- Experience level of nurses: new novice graduate nurse vs. expert nurse

- Nursing expertise, including but not limited to certifications, education

- Other disciplines or staff

- Technology

Ratio-based staffing has several potential issues. The first is that it is often based on RN-only ratios, leading administrators and managers to staff RNs to that level but cut other assistive staff levels back to manage the financial impact of a fixed ratio. The second is that hospital administrators may interpret the ratio as the maximum number of nurses needed, when on a given day, if acuity is taken into consideration, it is the minimum number of nurses needed. The third is that staffing by a ratio replaces minimally safe staffing for quality patient care and nursing judgment. Additionally, productive nursing hours used for ratios reported by a hospital may not be limited to direct patient care.

An additional issue regarding ratio numbers is that patient days might not average 24 hours. A patient for an elective surgery might arrive early on the admission day and depart late on the discharge day, resulting in a patient day of more than 24 hours. A study using a sample of hospitals from Pennsylvania found that patient days are, on average, about 10% longer than 24 hours (Spetz et al., 2008).

In ratio-based staffing, there is either a maximum number of patients to nurse or a minimum number of nurses per unit. In the situation where it is patient to nurse, no one nurse can be assigned more than a certain number of patients. Whereas in a unit-based ratio, the unit must have a specific number of nurses and patients, ratio-based staffing allows for some flexibility based on acuity or workload, for instance. One nurse on that unit could be assigned five patients who have less workload needs; another nurse on that unit could be assigned three patients who have higher work intensity. Overall, the average nurse to patient ratio may not exceed four patients per nurse as a unit average as an example.

Finance-Based Method: The Lagging Indicator

The *finance-based method* of staffing includes using historical data and evidence-based best practice staffing standards to build the most accurate predictive schedules, so that we are as prepared as possible to go in on any specific day with the resources that we need to take care of the patients that we anticipate based on data. Productivity will set a run rate over time, but there are many variables that influence productivity day to day that also need to be taken into consideration. Additionally, a metric such as productivity functions more as a control metric and has little to do with predictive analytics—thus why we call this method a *lagging indicator.*

In many situations, the finance department has budgeted a specific number of productive and nonproductive hours for your department based on past performance and historical patient trends. This is turned into a ratio for nurse staffing. So, how can this prepare you for day of operation?

Even if you've had the best planning possible as you get what you get right, you get the volumes you get, you get the staff skill mix that you get, and you can control for skill mix a little bit. But on any given day, you don't know when you're planning what your roster is going to look like:

- Are you going to have experienced nurses?

- Are you going to have a bunch of travelers?

- Are you going have a bunch of new grads on your roster?

So all of that impacts how you can affect your skill mix on day of operation. And once you get into day of operation, what productivity really represents is the decisions the charge nurse is making with the resources that they have because productivity is just a reflection of volume. Keep these guidelines in mind:

- If you have more experienced nurses, you might be able to use fewer resources.

- If the bulk of your staff is new grads, you might need more resources.
- If you have high-acuity patients, you might need less.
- If you have lower-acuity patients, you might need more.

There are so many factors on day of operation that impact your productivity that you need to use other methods such as acuity or workload intensity.

As a manager, you know you are responsible for your budget, and nurse staffing accounts for most of it. So, despite the limitations of finance-based methods, you will still need to be able to talk with the finance department. Knowledge is power, and although the finance department may hand you your unit's numbers on a weekly or monthly basis, you should know how to calculate your own numbers. If you were fortunate enough to read *The Nurse Manager's Guide to Budgeting & Finance*, 3rd Edition, you have seen Al Rundio's calculation of employee-related costs (2021). What follows are the calculations and explanations you need to know to be informed. It is important to note that the nurse manager determines the hours of care per patient per day to be budgeted based on standards of care that will lead to quality patient care.

The average daily census (ADC). To obtain this statistic, first add together census figures for each day in the given period. Then divide that total by the number of days.

Total census figures

÷ Total number of days

= ADC

The average monthly patient days. To obtain this number, include all days that patients (excluding newborns in the nursery) are hospitalized. The day of admission, but not the day of discharge, is counted as a patient day. If both admission and discharge occur the same day, the day is counted as one patient day. To obtain this statistic, multiply the average daily census by the number of days in the calendar year (365). Then divide the product of that calculation by the number of months in the year (12).

(ADC x 365) ÷ 12

= Average monthly patient days

The number of hours of nursing care to be provided. To obtain this number, multiply the total patient days per year by hours of care per patient day to be budgeted.

Total patient days per year

x Hours of care per patient per day

= Hours of nursing care to be provided

Skill mix—percentage of total nursing hours by skill. This is the percentage of hours worked by RNs, LPNs, nursing assistive personnel (NAPs), and contract staff by unit. To calculate this statistic, take the total number of hours worked by skill set in a specific unit (i.e., RN, LPN, NAP, or contract staff) and divide by total number of hours worked by staff with direct patient care responsibilities.

Total number of hours worked by skill (e.g., RN)

÷ Total number of hours worked by staff (hours of nursing care)

= Percentage of care provided by that skill

Nursing hours per patient day (NHPPD) is calculated by taking the total number of nursing staff providing care divided by the total number of patients in a given day.

NHPPD =

Total number of nursing staff on a given day

÷ Total number of patients in that same day

One challenge with using the calculated average, as demonstrated, is that it does not take into consideration that your unit's census today may be dramatically different from tomorrow's census. Here are some definitions you need to keep in mind:

- **Mean:** Most often referred to as average. Calculated by adding a group of numbers together and then dividing them by the total number of integers in that group.

- **Mode:** A set of numbers that occurs most often in a grouping of numbers. There may be no mode, one mode, or more than one mode.

- **Median:** In a set of numbers ordered from least to most, the median is the number right in the middle of that set.

NOTE

With a mean, large or small numbers will throw off the reliability of your data, leading to a smaller or larger mean or average than if you used the median. Using the median can correct for outliers.

Sometimes any one of these terms may be referred to as the "average." However, when you use any of these measures, what you are really looking at is the "measure of central tendency." The nature of the data drives whether you use one or the other. Makes sense, right? You want to know on any given day the central tendency of your census and staff needed. Depending on the type of unit and patient population, you may not want to use the mean but the median or mode instead.

Staffing for Patterns

As a young manager in the early 1990s, I did not have as many electronic tools or data available to me as there are today. I recognized that working on an OB unit, there seemed to be patterns of higher census. I manually calculated one-year patient days by days of the week on a four-week schedule that coincided with the four-week staff schedule. The pattern indicated that there were more patients during the third week of the staff schedule, which was valuable information.

The nurses worked eight-hour shifts at that time, with the exception of the few nurses who worked 12-hour shifts on the weekend. There were several nurses working a 0.5 full-time equivalent (FTE), which was one or two days the first week and three or four days on the second week of the pay period. I was then able to schedule a little heavier during that third week and on the days indicated by moving their days to that week of the schedule.

A second opportunity I discovered was that with the wide fluctuations in census, the mean, or average daily census, was rarely the actual number of patients present on the unit. I convinced my director to let me try staffing to the mode instead of the median. By doing so, there were more times that we had to staff down, but much time was saved by not scrambling for staff on a regular basis.

–Deborah Maust Martin, MBA, MSN, RN, NE-BC, FACHE

TIP

Just because the mean has always been used for staffing does not mean you need to use it. Calculate your mode and see what you get. Talk with your boss and ask to trial it. You both may be pleasantly surprised!

Chapter 1 discusses patient flow and variability. The key to variability is to manage it. Using the average or mean to schedule staff as you create the next cycle's schedule means you are probably treating each day as if the census does not change day to day, and you are left with wide fluctuations in staffing. Instead of managing your census variability, you are managing your staffing, the day of operations, shift by shift. In addition to your average census, two other census-driven data points are helpful in understanding your unit's needs for staffing and scheduling: core census and peak census. There are multiple ways to calculate these numbers, so, of course, see if your organization has a preferred definition first:

- **Core census:** the mean census of the lowest two months
- **Peak census:** the mean census of the highest two months

Knowing these numbers in addition to your average for all 12 months gives you a sense of potential issues around the low and high ends of your census, such as staff needing to take low census or higher float pool utilization to meet the needs of your patients.

Staffing and Scheduling: Electronic Programs

Staffing and scheduling nurses have typically not been evidence-based processes. They are complex and dynamic tasks that involve knowing what you need to staff in addition to how you will staff to provide quality patient care. Electronic programs are designed to help nurse managers move toward an evidence-based approach. There are two types of electronic programs for staffing:

- Those that assist with creating a schedule (getting nurses scheduled)
- Those that help you determine your staffing needs (how many nurses or personnel you need)

Some programs do both; others do one or the other. Despite the need to move toward an evidence-based approach, fewer than two-thirds of the hospitals in the United States have automated staffing and scheduling systems in place (Crist-Grundman & Mulrooney, 2011). The typical barriers are cost and competing priorities. A business case can be developed with the help of many of the vendors to demonstrate the positive financial and patient outcomes for purchasing and implementing an automated system.

Programs to Assist With Scheduling

Hospitals that have implemented software programs have found that an electronic scheduling system helps save time and money (Palmer, 2008). The more effective programs interface with payroll, leading to further cost savings. If your organization does not have an electronic program to maintain your schedule, we highly suggest that you work with your boss to present a case to purchase one. Scheduling systems are not cheap; however, a case can be built with a return on investment (ROI) for your organization. Your ROI will depend on your unique situation, such as how much you believe you can reduce casual labor costs and how much time will be saved in FTEs by obtaining this system. As you build that case, Table 2.1 includes items to consider.

TABLE 2.1   PROS AND CONS OF AN ELECTRONIC SCHEDULING SYSTEM

Pros	Cons
Decreased time spent calling staff to fill openings	Initial purchase costs and annual maintenance
Better utilization of pool/per diem staff	Need to standardize practices and processes across different units
Better management of various skills and competency	Organization may not be able to purchase additional modules to fully operationalize functionality that was given in initial demo
Better management of floating staff	Time needed to receive input and build system to match organization's needs
Reduction in contract labor	Centralization of staffing may mean actual and/or perceived loss of control by unit leadership
Staff empowerment to be a part of the process	Staff perspective on change in general; need to have good change-management process in place
Accuracy of electronic schedule	
Ability to move to a centralized staffing process	
Improved reporting mechanisms	

continues

TABLE 2.1   PROS AND CONS OF AN ELECTRONIC SCHEDULING SYSTEM   (CONT.)

Pros	Cons
Decreased time of higher paid staff to schedule	
Improved fairness to employees	
Transparency of all open shifts in an organization	

Implementing a New Staffing System

The challenging component of implementing a new scheduling and staffing system is the inclination to think of it as merely a new technology system, underestimating the emotional impact of any change to staff members' work schedules. Work is only one part of our lives, but work schedules can, or can be perceived to, significantly impact those things we value most—time with our families, social functions, self-care, finances, etc. On top of a "regular" work schedule, we often ask staff to do more and/or carry guilt for not being able to do more. Additionally, the stressors of work can insidiously infiltrate time away from work; I suspect few healthcare professionals are really able to walk out the door of the hospital and leave it all behind at the end of their shift. Implementing a new system needs to be weighted more on allowing staff involvement in design, listening to their concerns, and really understanding the impact of the changes prior to completing the plan for rollout.

–Vickie Whitham, MS, RN, NE-BC

Programs to Determine Staffing Needs

In addition to software programs to complete your staffing, programs can help determine what that staffing might be. These software programs take into consideration your patient population and can be individualized for it, or you can use the formulas the company has predeveloped. Often, these programs have proprietary methods that will assist you in accounting for differences in patients' requirements for nursing care. Based on how you decide to input the data into the software program (manually or by interfacing with your EHR), you can get data to inform staffing your unit hour by hour or shift by shift.

As with other systems, using a staffing software program has benefits and potential issues, as noted in Table 2.2. Because many automated systems are based on acuity and work intensity, the pros and cons of using such a system may also include those listed earlier in Table 2.1.

TABLE 2.2   ADVANTAGES AND DISADVANTAGES TO STAFFING SOFTWARE

Advantages	Disadvantages
Real-time documentation by nurses	Cost
Standardized approach shift to shift	Time to develop
Data to tie to outcomes and budget	Time to maintain, including reliability testing
Transparency of true needs for all units	Organization not purchasing all the modules and getting the basic program with limited functionality
Evidence-based decision-making to staff	
Improved collaboration with staff	
Improved patient outcomes due to managing appropriate staffing levels (research noted in Chapter 1)	

Fixed, Self-Scheduling, and Rotating Schedules

Whether you go with an electronic scheduling system or use pen and paper, you need to decide whether to use a fixed schedule or to let the staff self-schedule. A *fixed schedule* is one in which Nurse A always works Monday, Tuesday, and Wednesday, and Nurse B always works Thursday, Friday, and Saturday, for instance. *Self-scheduling* is when you allow nurses to schedule themselves after you post a schedule of open shifts. Finally, there is the *rotating schedule*, where some aspects of the schedule may be fixed, but there is a set rotation for the staff. This rotation may include days to nights, for example.

In some places, staff members may turn in their dream schedules, and the manager develops the schedule based on that information. Talk about time-consuming. Of all the types of scheduling, self-scheduling is backed by research that demonstrates improved nurse satisfaction rates (Beltzhoover, 1994; Robb et al., 2003).

However, there are benefits and downfalls to all three methods, as noted in Tables 2.3, 2.4, and 2.5.

TABLE 2.3   ADVANTAGES AND DISADVANTAGES TO FIXED SCHEDULES

Advantages	Disadvantages
Staff members always know their schedules	May interrupt staff members' lives
Can provide continuity for patient care	Recruiting new employees may become difficult
Some staff prefer fixed shifts	Staff members on fixed schedules become a mini-culture unto themselves
Unbalanced skill mixes can be fixed	Increased turnover as newer nurses have to work many years to advance into perceived better schedules

TABLE 2.4   ADVANTAGES AND DISADVANTAGES TO SELF-SCHEDULING

Advantages	Disadvantages
Staff has increased control and flexibility	There are no guaranteed times
Number of change requests decreases	Staff waits until last minute to schedule, not meeting FTE
Manager spends less time scheduling	Continuity of patient care decreases if staff is not scheduled back to back for shifts
Schedule fits staff's personal life	It is difficult to manage right skill mix for each shift
Absenteeism decreases	

TABLE 2.5   ADVANTAGES AND DISADVANTAGES TO ROTATING SCHEDULES

Advantages	Disadvantages
All staff has equal chance to work day shift	Staff does prefer fixed or self-scheduling over rotating
Maximize staff skill mix	Health problems increase
Educational costs decrease by rotating staff through training	Well-being decreases

When determining which method to use, make sure you get staff input! This is their schedule, their life. Research has shown that self-scheduling results in improved staff satisfaction, improved quality of care, and better work life balance, among many outcomes (Wynendaele et al., 2021).

Summary

Here are the key points covered in this chapter:

- It is important to know what your organization says about staffing because it may have compiled the research and made recommendations to take into consideration.

- Staffing levels for registered nurses and other staff should meet at least those required by state, accreditation, institutional, and professional guidelines including patient needs.

- Using only one method to determine staffing will not meet the needs of patients.

- Staffing for quality needs to consider current patient census and acuity, work intensity, nursing time and interventions, length of stay, skill mix, expertise of staff, and nonpatient care time.

- Routine evaluation of staffing impact on patient outcomes needs to be completed, and adjustments to staffing should be made.

References

American Nurses Association. (2021). *Nursing: Scope and standards of practice* (4th ed.). Author.

American Nurses Association. (2023). *Advocating for safe staffing.* https://www.nursingworld.org/practice-policy/nurse-staffing/nurse-staffing-advocacy/

Association of Women's Health, Obstetric and Neotatal Nurses. (2021). *Standards for professional registered nurse staffing for perinatal units.* https://www.awhonn.org/education/staffing-exec-summary/

Beltzhoover, M. (1994). Self-scheduling: An innovative approach. *Nurse Manager, 25*(4), 81–82.

California Department of Public Health. (2008). *Changes to the minimum licensed nurse to patient ratios effective January 1, 2008.* https://www.cdph.ca.gov/Programs/CHCQ/LCP/Pages/AFL-07-26.aspx

Centers for Medicare & Medicaid Services. (2010). *Code of federal regulations. Title 42: Public health.* https://www.gpo.gov/fdsys/pkg/CFR-2011-title42-vol5/pdf/CFR-2011-title42-vol5.pdf

Centers for Medicare & Medicaid Services. (2023). *Medicare and Medicaid programs: Minimum staffing standards for long-term care facilities and Medicaid institutional payment transparency reporting.* https://www.cms.gov/newsroom/fact-sheets/medicare-and-medicaid-programs-minimum-staffing-standards-long-term-care-facilities-and-medicaid

Crist-Grundman, D., & Mulrooney, G. (2011). Effective workforce management starts with leveraging technology, while staffing optimization requires true collaboration. *Nursing Economic$, 29*(4), 195–200.

Dall'Ora, C., Ejebu, O.-Z., Ball, J., & Griffiths, P. (2023). Shift work characteristics and burnout among nurses: Cross-sectional survey. *Occupational Medicine, 73*(4), 199–204. https://doi.org/10.1093/occmed/kqad046

Department of Human Services. (2023). *Hospital staffing procedures and requirements to comply with HB 2697.* https://www.oregon.gov/oha/PH/RULESREGULATIONS/Documents/PH_59-2023TrackedChanges.pdf

Moore, E. C., Tolley, C. L., Bates, D. W., & Slight, S. P. (2020). A systematic review of the impact of health information technology on nurses' time. *Journal of the American Medical Informatics Association, 27*(5), 798–807. https://doi.org/10.1093/jamia/ocz231

Palmer, A. (2008, February). Right on schedule. *Incentive Magazine, 182*(2), 38–40.

Rerkjirattikal, P., Huynh, V.-N., Olapiriyakul, S., & Supnithi, T. (2020). A goal programming approach to nurse scheduling with individual preference satisfaction. *Mathematical Problems in Engineering, 2020*(1), 1–11. https://doi.org/10.1155/2020/2379091

Robb, E. A., Determan, A. C., Lampat, L. R., Scherbring, M. J., Slifka, R. M., & Smith, N. A. (2003). Self-scheduling: Satisfaction guaranteed? *Nurse Manager, 34*(7), 16–18.

Rundio, A. (2021). *The nurse manager's guide to budgeting & finance* (3rd ed.). Sigma Theta Tau International.

Skinner, M. (n.d.). A guide to mandatory overtime for nurses. *IntelyCare*. https://www.intelycare.com/career-advice/a-guide-to-mandatory-overtime-for-nurses

Spetz, J., Donaldson, N., Aydin, C., & Brown, D. S. (2008). How many nurses per patient? Measurements of nurse staffing in health services research. *Health Services Research, 43*(5 Pt. 1), 1674–1692. https://doi.org/10.1111/j.1475-6773.2008.00850.x

Stimpfel, A. W., Sloane, D. M., & Aiken, L. H. (2012). The longer the shifts for hospital nurses, the higher the levels of burnout and patient dissatisfaction. *Health Affairs, 31*(11), 2501–2509. https://doi.org/10.1377/hlthaff.2011.1377

Washington State Nurses Association. (2023). *New Oregon law establishes safe staffing ratios.* https://www.wsna.org/news/2023/new-oregon-law-establishes-safe-staffing-ratios#:~:text=11%2C%202023.-,On%20Aug.,to%20put%20ratios%20into%20statute

Wynendaele, H., Gemmel, P., Pattyn, E., Myny, D., & Trybou, J. (2021). Systematic review: What is the impact of self-scheduling on the patient, nurse and organization? *Journal of Advanced Nursing, 77*(1), 47–82. https://doi.org/10. 1111/jan.14579

PART 2

Researching & Operating Safe Staffing Principles and Practices

Start With Understanding Your Unit's Care Delivery Model

We have all heard, "This is the way we have always done it." Surprisingly, we still hear this today. We have all been at meetings where someone brought up a new idea, and the immediate response was something like: "We are fine, we don't need to change," or, "That is not how we do it here," which is code for, "This is the way we have always done it, and it's not going to change!" Do you sit back and think to yourself, "At least I contributed today," or, "I tried"? But did you? Did you stop at the pushback, or did you push back on the pushback your received? What if you had added, "True, but we all know those who fail to evolve eventually become extinct"?

We open with this scenario because we want you to think differently about staffing. We want you to challenge the status quo. Doing something new or different always requires change management, and nurse managers do not get much education on that. In a study conducted in 2023, the biggest challenge organizations face is a lack of change management expertise among leaders (Healthcare Plus Solutions Group, 2023). As a nurse manager, you will need to manage the change both for those who want to change with you and for those who do not want to change. Failing to manage change on your unit could lead to a failure to successfully change at all.

> **TIP**
>
> *A famous leadership quote is "culture eats strategy for lunch," by Dr. Peter Drucker. If you don't understand the relationship between your unit's culture and your change or "strategy," it will always be at risk for failure. Managing change means managing and leading your unit's culture. As noted at the beginning of this chapter, reflect on the true driver for changing your care delivery model. Whatever the reason, ensure that your unit or department's staff are at the table to help create it. Do not just tell them what they will be doing.*

This chapter discusses what we traditionally call models of care, the impact they may have on staffing, and the approaches to resource support you need to consider. We challenge you to understand the past and present and to create new future models.

Care Delivery Models

In the post-COVID-19 era, it seems like everyone is talking about new care delivery models, particularly as a way to staff during this latest nurse shortage. However, every "new" model we have heard nurses talk about has been around for decades. There really isn't anything brand-new—maybe just new to you or slight variations of what already existed. As you or your hospital consider new care delivery models, keep in close consideration that systems of nursing care delivery are a reflection of social values, management ideology, and economic considerations and have continued to evolve since the 1930's (Tiedeman & Lookinland, 2004). So much of today's conversation around care delivery models is really about staffing and scheduling, driven by economic considerations and not so much about true innovative care delivery that reflects societal values of care.

As the nurse manager, you get to manage and lead your unit to great patient outcomes. And we want you to continue that charge! Nursing care delivery models are ways of organizing and delivering patient care. How you structure patient care and who performs that care should be at the heart of any care delivery model. Typically, when we think of care delivery models, we consider factors like whom you staff and how you staff. However, that still feels like staffing and scheduling and not really a care delivery model. Moving the chairs around the proverbial deck isn't going to result in new outcomes anytime soon.

In the following pages, we discuss various traditional care delivery models. As the nurse manager, seek permission to change or pilot a new-to-you care delivery model. Different care delivery models may have a positive or negative impact on your budget, but so do adverse patient outcomes. Take the time to meet with your finance department and explain what you would like to do. On paper, figure out different models with the staff needed and associated costs. Think of your current budget. If you do not exceed your current budget, it shouldn't matter how you use that budgeted money to provide care. If you exceed your budget, you may be able to offset the increase in costs with improved patient outcomes and/or decreased nurse turnover.

TIP

Often true innovation is stifled as finance and hospital executives continue to want data points for comparison. Hours per patient day, productive and nonproductive time, as well as the staffing mix among other indicators may have to look drastically different if we really want to change how care is delivered. With anything new, there will not be any comparator benchmarks! You may have to meet regularly with finance to determine what new measures may be appropriate. Many of us have been told to be innovative, yet are held to traditional finance and nurse productivity measures that constrain true innovation as the measurements of the past models may no longer be relevant.

There are many definitions of traditional care delivery, whether you are discussing a unit, a hospital, a community, or a nation. At each of these levels, the care delivery model looks very different, because the goals are very different at different levels. The unit and organization have the most direct impact on the patient and outcomes today. Added complexity leads to different care delivery models even within the same organization, which is acceptable. It would not make sense for the medical-surgical unit, for example, to be structured like the labor and delivery unit, which has different nursing care requirements with different goals for patient care. When thinking about your care delivery model, you should consider four main components. The model should:

- **Have a consistent and standardized structure.** Each shift, each day, every unit-based staff member and float nurse will be able to rely on the same structure without trying to figure out on each shift what they should be doing related to patient care. Staff can rely on coming to work to provide primary care or team-based care, as opposed to switching frequently from one care delivery model to another. If your model changes, then it really is a staffing model, not a care delivery model!

- **Have accountability and responsibility in its structure.** No matter your model, ensure that the nurses know who is accountable, what each person is responsible for, and whom they report to through the chain of command. If there are problems for staffing or patient care, do they know whom they can reach out to immediately to help them resolve an issue?

- **Provide organization to the rules and structure in policies, procedures, or guidelines.** Educate your staff on these, and ensure that your staff knows the scope of practice for each person on the unit as well as what can be delegated. Inability to delegate or lack of confidence in delegation will hamper a team- or function-based model.

- **Define how work is organized, define how staff is deployed, and explain who does what in providing patient care.** This can best be accomplished through pictorial models and job descriptions. A picture that demonstrates the care delivery model serves as a quick reference for chain of command and clarifying the work relationship between members of your care delivery model. Include trust and mutual understanding of roles, skills, and responsibilities.

In addition to appropriate delegation, nurses need to feel comfortable that what they are delegating is within the education, training, and competence of that individual, licensed or not. Having a transparent education record may be useful so that staff can quickly determine whether someone can appropriately carry out a delegated intervention. If there is no transparency, nurses may be hesitant to delegate, again hampering your care delivery model from functioning correctly.

In reviewing what you want in your care delivery model, think first about a consistent and standardized structure. Do you want to manage and staff a care delivery model where the main components are different day to day, shift to shift? If you have a different mix of nurses and staff every shift—RNs, LPNs, and nursing assistive personnel (NAPs)—then you do not have any one care delivery model. For example, you might have an all-RN staff today, and tomorrow you have an all-RN staff plus one LPN on the unit. How can you have a primary care model with an LPN? Do you or your staff treat the LPN like an RN? Or how about those days when you are so short you will take anything, including more NAPs, because you cannot get enough RNs? If this describes your unit in any way, your care delivery model is inconsistent and not standardized. You may need to focus on roster management. In this scenario, you do not have reliability in your model and will force staff members to become task-oriented as staff abilities change shift to shift. You may find you get outcomes that are inconsistent as well as staff members who are confused about their own roles in providing care.

Here are some questions to ask yourself regarding your care delivery components:

- Is each member functioning at the top of their license?

- Are there organizational barriers such as policies that are artificially limiting the RNs' and others' scope of practice?

- Are you clear regarding what you are accountable and responsible for? How about your staff?

- Does the shift feel calm even when busy (organized), or does each shift feel frenzied and rushed (chaotic)?

- Are you and your staff members clear on how patient care is organized among them and other disciplines, or does it seem like staff is duplicating efforts or some tasks are not getting done each day?

- Does each person understand their role, the skills of others, and responsibilities to the whole team?

- Are these components clearly defined in your current care delivery model?

Using these components, how would you structure your staff and care differently? As mentioned in Chapter 1 with value-based care and Accountable Care Organizations (ACOs), the care delivery models we have today will be insufficient to meet the outcomes in tomorrow's healthcare environment. For some of you, maybe that tomorrow is today. The following sections will help you understand the various care delivery models that may work for you, including team, modular, primary, and functional nursing.

Team-Based Nursing

Team-based nursing is the concept of RNs, LPNs, and NAPs (such as nursing assistants) working together to identify, plan, implement, and evaluate patient-centered care. The key concept is that the team works together toward comprehensive nursing care. Different types of personnel can meet the goal of team nursing, including the RN, LPN, *and* NAP. Your goal as a nurse manager is to ensure that the care of the patient is distributed among these team members to accomplish the plan of care. The goal is to increase the involvement of the RN in planning and coordinating care and delegating interventions as appropriate. The benefits and potential issues of team nursing are described in Table 3.1.

TABLE 3.1   BENEFITS AND POTENTIAL ISSUES OF TEAM NURSING

Benefits	Potential Issues
Overall unit staff costs less	RN does not delegate appropriately
Attitude of "it's not my patient" decreases	Workload is not distributed evenly
Opportunity for mentoring increases	Lack of communication can be detrimental
Leadership skills of RN in team increase	Patients may be uncomfortable or confused with multiple caregivers

Staff RN's Experience With Team Nursing

During my last month working as an RN in the labor and delivery unit of a busy suburban hospital, we had occasion to experience team nursing at its finest. The shift began like any other; my very sweet patient was in labor with her second child, and her pain was intensifying. The patient refused an epidural, stating that she had one during her first labor and it was ineffective. Eventually the pain became too much, and the patient changed her mind. Within 20 minutes of her request, the patient's epidural was placed by the anesthesiologist, but something was obviously wrong. Within 10 minutes of completion of the procedure, the patient stopped breathing, and the fetal heart tones dropped considerably. The epidural medication had migrated up the epidural space as opposed to down and had paralyzed the patient's diaphragm. This required the baby to be delivered while the patient was unconscious and being ventilated with a bag and mask.

It was amazing to have a capable and organized RN team leader who responded to my call out immediately and mobilized a group that included the anesthesiologist, the OB/GYN, several RNs, and ancillary staff members who assisted in the rapid delivery of the baby and reversal of the patient's epidural. I had worked more than 14 years in this role and had never experienced this particular patient situation. The fact that the patient suffered respiratory arrest not only was quite alarming but could have easily been disastrous had my team leader and coworkers not mobilized so quickly and been competent and willing to help.

–Toni Tanzella, MSN, FNP

Outcomes related to team nursing are inconsistent across studies; however, these outcomes are no different than when compared to other nursing care delivery models (Beckett et al., 2021). However, it has been consistently noted that it is imperative to educate your staff on delegation so that this model of care can be successful (Beckett et al., 2021). Nurses with ineffective delegation skills may have a negative impact on patient safety (Magnusson et al., 2017).

Modular Nursing

Modular nursing is a modification of team nursing, where there is a greater focus on the patient's geographic location for staff assignment (Yoder-Wise, 2003). In this model, the unit is divided into pods, or modules, with the same consistent RNs, LPNs, and/or NAPs assigned to work together within those pods. As evidence-based hospital design continues to advance and is incorporated into facilities, components of this nursing care delivery model will already be incorporated by design. If your hospital is older or has not incorporated evidence-based design, then this model may be beneficial to you. The space in which care is provided has a major impact on nurse productivity. Think about the time it takes nurses on your unit to walk and get needed supplies and see all their patients. Does it take time away from patient care? This model could improve your unit's productivity. Table 3.2 describes the benefits and potential issues of modular nursing.

TABLE 3.2   BENEFITS AND POTENTIAL ISSUES OF MODULAR NURSING

Benefits	Potential Issues
RN has opportunities for leadership development	Staff may create subcultures on your unit
RN focuses on planning and coordination	Stocking each area with necessary patient care supplies increases costs
Communication is more efficient	Not all hospital structures are conducive to this care model
Staff saves time through geographical closeness	

Primary Nursing

Primary nursing is the model of care delivery in which an RN (usually teamed with a nursing assistant) provides all the care that cannot be delegated to the assistant to a small group of patients. Traditional versions of the primary nursing model suggested that the primary RN was accountable for care 24 hours a day from admission to discharge (you might consider this version in an ACO); however, the current model assigns accountability only for the length of the shift the RN is working. This shift occurred with the movement towards 12-hour shifts decreasing consistency of staff over any one patient's admission coupled with a shorter length of stay for most patients.

The primary nursing model is typically the most expensive model, as it uses the most RNs (the highest-paid caregivers on the team), leading to higher RN hours per patient day. Some research does show improved patient satisfaction levels with primary nursing compared with other models of care (Tonkikh et al., 2020). Additionally, research has noted a shorter length of stay for patients in a primary care model (Chen et al., 2020).

To determine whether this model would be cost-effective for your unit, look at your quality data, such as pressure ulcers and falls, and hospital-acquired infections, such as pneumonia. Based on the research, with an increase in RN staff, how much money would be offset in improved outcomes? Table 3.3 describes further benefits and potential issues of primary nursing.

TABLE 3.3   BENEFITS AND POTENTIAL ISSUES OF PRIMARY NURSING

Benefits	Potential Issues
Limited number of caregivers for the patient	Higher staff costs
Improved nursing-sensitive patient outcomes	RN dissatisfaction with providing all care
Increased autonomy	Limited ability to build delegation skills
Improved skill development (self-reliance)	Failure of RN to ask for help when needed
Strengthened nurse-patient relationship	Uneven patient assignments

Functional Nursing

The *functional nursing* care delivery model has a task-oriented focus, in which different standards of the nursing scope of practice are assigned to each staff member. To complete the care needed for all the unit's patients, RNs and other personnel are assigned various tasks. This could include assigning an LPN to pass all medications; an RN to complete all admissions, discharges, and transfers; and a nursing assistant to give all the baths. The charge nurse or manager usually decides who gets which tasks after considering team members' strengths and weaknesses. Typically, you see this in non–acute care facilities where there are fewer RNs and a greater number of LPNs and NAPs.

This model for the acute care setting has more potential issues than benefits. Table 3.4 describes the further benefits and potential issues of functional nursing.

TABLE 3.4   BENEFITS AND POTENTIAL ISSUES OF FUNCTIONAL NURSING

Benefits	Potential Issues
Lower staffing costs	Fragmented care
Large amount of work completed quickly	Task-oriented or technical nurses
Quick learning process for how to perform tasks	Decreased RN accountability and responsibility
Improve knowledge, skill, and ability in those repetitively assigned tasks	Diminished RN-patient relationship
	Poor evaluation and documentation of nursing care
	No one person has all answers regarding patient care
	Increased risk for errors due to increased speed of completing tasks

In addition to a unit care delivery model, there are organization and system-level care delivery models. The unit and organizational models should not compete but rather complement each other. Multiple models can exist, as each unit and organization is unique. What model does your organization follow? Here are some examples of organizational care delivery models:

- 12-bed hospital
- Virtual ICU and virtual med-surg
- Primary care team
- Transitional care model
- Hospital at home
- ACOs
- Medical or health homes

Additional Support Teams

In addition to understanding your care delivery model, what other types of nursing support services do you have or need? Throughout this book, we look at other nursing and non-nursing support and resources. These next sections describe the float pool and rapid response team. Both can have positive impacts on your care delivery model. Knowing that you have additional backup resources for your unit allows you to make informed decisions as you determine your staffing needs and prepare the schedule.

Float Pools

This type of resource has many names. Whether you call these nurses *float pool*, *per diem*, or *resource team*, all perform about the same function for the organization: fill in schedule and staffing gaps as they arise. Although the float pool may not be a "unit" in the traditional sense, float pool staff members are a unit as a group of nurses and have their own culture. Float pools should supply nurses to units to meet staffing needs in these situations:

1. Illness or bereavement leave

2. Coverage for a period with higher-than-normal vacation requests

3. FMLA and maternity/paternity leave

4. Short-term coverage during unexpected turnover

Float pools should not be expected to provide ongoing staff coverage for chronically understaffed units. Unit managers monitor and hire based on their roster needs (Chapter 11) in order to most effectively manage full-time equivalents (FTE), plan coverage for various leaves of absence, plan ahead for planned turnover (i.e., your RNs graduating and becoming nurse practitioners), and forecast hiring needs.

If your organization does not have a robust float/per diem team, your unit-based RNs may be floated to cover shortages in other units. For many, floating a unit-based RN outside their specialty can cause anxiety, stress, disruption, and dissatisfaction. Floating staff RNs in this manner is a short-term solution to your scheduling and staffing and roster management issues. When unit-based RNs are floated to an area outside their specialty, such as an orthopedic nurse to a medical unit, the organization is reinforceing that nurses do not have specific bodies of knowledge based on that specific patient population. This reinforces a misperception that RNs work is task-based and not knowledge-based. This method should be reserved for disaster and emergency management only.

As healthcare, nursing, and medicine advance, nurses can become as specialized in different areas of practice (thus certification!) as physicians in specialty practices. It is important to note that it takes a certain type of nurse to be a successful float nurse; they must learn multiple areas of specialty care to remain competent in all units in which they practice. Floating should be considered a specialty. You should pay appropriate attention to hiring and training nurses who are a good match for this type of work. If you do not have a consistent care delivery model with role clarity, nurses or other staff members who float to your unit are liable to make errors as they struggle to figure out their roles in providing patient care on your unit.

TIP

Having consistent unit-based staff is important for positive patient outcomes. A unit should strive to have no more than 10% to 20% of its daily staffing needs met by float or per diem nurses. Although float staff do maintain competency in multiple areas, your unit-based RNs are the experts for your patient population.

Having a dedicated float pool has several benefits and potential issues, as noted in Table 3.5.

TABLE 3.5   BENEFITS AND POTENTIAL ISSUES OF A DEDICATED FLOAT POOL

Benefits	Potential Issues
Increases staff morale and satisfaction	Masks issue of higher turnover rates
Decreases turnover of dedicated floor staff	Unit-based staff may not get all hours in to meet FTE requirements before float staff is used
Decreases potential for adverse events	Increases education costs for maintaining education across many specialties
Maintains specialization of nurses to their unit specialty	Treats float staff like outsiders or gives unfair assignments
Decreases costs from fewer premium labor or shift incentives	Easier for poorly performing RNs to "hide"

Two questions typically arise when considering whether to use a float pool:

1. How many RNs (or other types of staff) do we need in a float pool?

2. What type of RN is best for this position?

To figure the number of float RNs (or other staff) that may be needed, as well as your potential cost savings, you will need to look at your unit's and hospital's information as follows:

1. Review data from a specific time period, preferably six months to one year. If there was a significant practice change that could affect the numbers, start after that change. You can annualize numbers if you believe the time period will remain an accurate reflection.

2. Identify the total number of hours used for traveling and registry RNs, RN overtime, and RN incentive pay (your organization may or may not have incentive pay, and there may be some overlap in these dollar amounts, such as a travel RN who also gets overtime).

3. Determine the total number of dollars spent in each of those three categories. (If you do not use a category, obviously you will not include it.)

4. Divide the total number of hours used by 1,872 (0.9 full-time RN working three 12-hour shifts a week/52 weeks a year). The result will be the number of full-time equivalents (FTEs) used. Use this number as the basis for the number of float staff you and your organization may need.

    Total hours used by RN traveler, overtime, and incentive pay

    ÷ 1,872

    = Total number 0.9 FTEs needed

5. Divide the total number of hours from step 2 by the total amount spent in step 3 to determine the average wage you are paying.

In looking at the final number, is there a cost savings? Typically, a float RN makes less than the combination of traveler pay, incentive pay, and overtime. So, take the number from step 4 and multiply it by the expected hourly wage of your float RN before overtime (not a traveler RN, registry RN, overtime, or incentive pay). Multiply this by 1,872. Then subtract this number from step 3. This is your *potential* cost savings. Here's the formula:

Total number of FTEs needed

x average hourly wage of a float RN

x 1,872

− number from step 3

= total amount spent on travel and registry RNs, overtime, and incentive pay = potential cost savings

NOTE

Although you will not be able to reduce all overtime and incentive pay, you may be able to eliminate all travelers. In a few exceptions, this might not be a cost savings if you are very good at utilizing your current resources!

Next, how do you determine how many FTEs are needed to float to each area? When figuring the hours for step 2, you should pull these numbers by unit. If you divide the unit number by 1,872, you will get the number of FTEs for that unit. Now add up all like type units. The reason you want to break this out at a unit level is to determine the specialty areas that need the most and least help. If you need the most help in the emergency department (ED) but hire mostly RNs who are experienced floating to medical-surgical units and telemetry, you will spend more time orienting them. You would rather hire experienced ED nurses to fill the need and then teach them to float in other areas with less demand when your organization has the ability to do so. Here's the formula:

Total number of hours used for traveling RNs, registry RNs, RN overtime, and RN incentive pay

÷ 1,872

= number of FTEs needed in float pool

> ***TIP***
>
> *Do not treat your float pool as a solution for poor nurse retention. This will still l ead to poor staff and patient satisfaction as well as poor patient outcomes. If you have poor nurse satisfaction or high turnover, get to the root of the issue and fix it. The float pool should be there only to help out on an infrequent basis. In low-census months, float pool might be 10% of your unit's staffing, while in high-volume months, it may increase to 15% to 20% of your unit's staffing. Note that your float pool needs may also fluctuate related to your RN turnover rates.*

In determining your float pool, here are the critical business questions you should be asking:

- **Do you have enough core resources?** That is, does your unit have a dedicated staff so that you do not have a high float-pool utilization?

- **How do you ensure that your float RNs are scheduled to their commitments?** This ensures that with your regular staff you will meet your unit's scheduling needs.

- **Are float RNs benefited FTEs or not?** The preference is not, as you will increase your fixed expenses. Not having benefits decreases fixed costs—therefore, the reason you pay them a higher rate.

- **Will there be a gradual pay increase for committing to more shifts per month?** This increases your ability to cover more holes in your schedule with a dedicated float-pool RN.

- **Who will do their evaluations and monitor their practice?** Consistent evaluations and expectations will increase the comfort level of you and your staff when float nurses work in your unit, knowing that these RNs are just as capable as other RNs on your unit.

- **What will you pay them?** Do you pay enough to incentivize them to work in this unit and to compensate them for the skill of floating? This will increase the likelihood of more covered holes in your schedule.

- **Will you promise a certain amount of work, or will there be no guarantee of any hours?** If you have no guarantee of hours, some RNs may work at multiple organizations to ensure they get enough hours, which may decrease their day-to-day availability to you to fill in your schedule.

- **Will you expect availability for a minimum number of shifts per month?** Expecting a minimum number will give you an idea of how many shifts you can count on from the float pool to cover unmet scheduling needs on your unit.

- **Will you pay float staff holiday, weekend, and night premiums?** Paying premiums like the regular staff get will increase the likelihood that float staff may work more than minimum expectations, again contributing to increased help when you need it.

Float pools provide flexibility in your organization to meet staffing demands as census fluctuates. Float nurses are typically also more cost-effective than travel RNs, registry RNs, and overtime for your own staff. Having a proper size float pool will give your organization appropriate coverage to help you ensure safe staffing levels. Next, we discuss rapid response teams and their impact on your unit.

Rapid Response Teams

A *rapid response team* (RRT), *high-acuity response team* (HART), or *medical emergency team* is typically a team of healthcare providers, such as a mix of physician and/or advanced practice nurse (NP or CNS), RN, and respiratory therapist, who respond to high-acuity cases to decrease the risk of further deterioration, such as a cardiac or respiratory arrest. RRTs are invaluable to hospital and nursing staff. Often these teams focus on medical patients; however, with a shortage of behavioral health beds, there are more psychiatry or behavioral health RRTs.

> ### Consider This
>
> Whereas some patients will deteriorate despite the best clinical care, some patients deteriorate because of inadequate, missed, or delayed care, which includes clinician training and/or appropriate level of staffing to meet the level of care needed by that patient for that patient's condition (Litvak & Pronovost, 2010). Track and trend RRT usage to ensure that your unit and hospital are getting to the appropriate root cause of RRT use, which may be wholly patient-related and cannot always be controlled, as opposed to things like staffing and training that we do control.

When looking at the support services for your unit, take into consideration the support the RRT can give your staff. Multiple studies have demonstrated positive outcomes with the implementation of an RRT; however, results are varied, which could be a result of inadequate staffing (Zhang et al., 2024).

RRTs can be staffed with personnel that have another primary responsibility during the shift; however, for many, this is their primary assignment. For efficiency, most hospitals do not have a dedicated team (and we hope no hospital has so many calls that it requires a dedicated team). Although a secondary job with the RRT is just as important as the staff member's primary job, providing staffing for both the RRT and patient care assignment can be a difficult task.

One way to maintain productivity of the nurse on an RRT is to have that nurse work in a non–direct care RN position, such as an admission, discharge, or transfer (ADT) nurse or the resource or stat nurse for that shift. That way, if the nurse is pulled to an RRT, they will not urgently leave a patient assignment. Another method is to use an ICU nurse during the day without an assignment and use an ICU nurse at night who has a light assignment, such as one stable ICU patient whose care could be transferred to another nurse immediately.

Here are some items to consider for your schedule and staffing if you do not have an RRT:

- **Do you have an expert nurse on each shift?** There should be a resource on each shift who has the experience and competence to assist your newer nurses. Night shift tends to have more new graduate RNs and fewer resources than day shift. Ensure that the schedule has an expert each night to help triage and assist if a patient starts to deteriorate.

- **How many novice or new grad RNs should one shift have?** With the nursing shortage, you may not be able to prevent having several newer nurses on any one shift. But you can have a plan in place where expert nurses help the newer nurses better manage their patient load in addition to providing a mentored experience.

- **What are the resources on night shift for RNs?** There are typically fewer managers, educators, and advanced practice RNs on night shift, if any. Make sure it is clear to your staff whom to call and who their resources are after hours. Although you may have an administrative supervisor on during nights, typically they are very busy and may not be able to help immediately. Schedule resources, such as the educator, to occasionally flex to night shift to assess and work with newer staff during the shift.

- **How do you match novice RNs with more experienced RNs as a resource?** After precepting is finished, consider partnering your novice or newer RNs with more experienced RNs in a mentorship relationship. It is helpful if they are on the same shift; however, the connection between the two is most important for a successful partnership. Staff members who do not have the same resources as the day shift will appreciate this additional support.

- **Is the charge RN accessible to novice RNs during the shift?** If each night-charge nurse takes a patient load, they will not always be ready to help the newer or novice RN. Charge RNs should be able to round on all patients and be ready to help with staff RNs' patients as the need arises without compromising the care of their own patient loads. This is also a great opportunity to build the skills of those newer or novice RNs at night.

- **Have the charge RNs been given the time in their shift to mentor all staff?** Consider the role of the charge RN on both night and day shifts. As you plan the care delivery model and staff your unit, take into consideration the leadership role the charge nurse plays in leading and teaching your RNs on that shift.

RRTs should provide an additional layer to assist your staff, particularly your more novice staff, in taking care of emergent issues before they become critical.

Internationally Educated Nurses

Over the last several decades, the United States and other high-income nations have turned increasingly toward internationally educated nurse (IEN) recruitment to fill gaps in their nursing workforce. Organizations have been relying on IENs to fill in staffing gaps as early as 2002, when in fact, organizations needed to address the work environment and pay for the current nurses. Not much has changed over the last two decades! So much work to improve work environments has gone untouched, hoping that IENs will be willing to work in poor work environments.

This has been a controversial topic on many fronts, as it is an issue of freedom to migrate as well as an issue of distributive justice and social accountability. In 2010, the World Health Organization (WHO) published the Global Code of Practice on the International Recruitment of Health Personnel. The code sets the ethical norms and principles that were adopted by the World Health Assembly (WHA) in 2010 and urges member states to train and retain the health personnel they need, thereby limiting demand for international migration, especially from the understaffed health systems in low- and middle-income countries.

Fast forward to 2022, the WHO Global Code of Practice on the International Recruitment of Health Personnel report noted that 15% of healthcare workers globally are working outside of their country of birth. The Health Workforce Support and Safeguards List developed in 2020 consists of 47 countries. These countries face the most pressing health workforce challenges related to a very low density of doctors, nurses, and midwives that is below the global median (i.e., 48.6 per 10,000 population). The WHO has stated that this number has now increased to 55 countries requiring priority support for health workforce development and health system strengthening, along with additional safeguards that limit active international recruitment. Any recruitment from these 55 countries should (WHO, 2022):

- Be informed by health labor market analysis and the adoption of measures to ensure adequate supply of health workers in the source countries

- Engage Ministries of Health in the negotiation and implementation of agreements

- Specify the health system benefits of the arrangement to both source and destination countries

The ethics involved require a balance between the right to the highest attainable standard of health for source country populations and the right of health personnel to migrate (WHO, 2010). However, recruitment of IENs should not be a remedy for a continuously poor work environment. Not enough can be stated that US-based organizations should prioritize improving their work environment for all employees to attract and retain local staff. If an organization is having issues with retaining staff due to a poor working environment that native-born nurses will not accept, why would it be acceptable to allow IENs to practice in that environment?

Poor work environments and nurse burnout are experienced by nurses in all countries. The US has continued to recruit from the Philippines, falsely believing that they have extra nurses. In the Philippines, burnout is leading to an unstaffed healthcare system, which faces a shortage of 127,000 nurses itself (Lalu, 2023). Unfortunately, nurse burnout is a universal issue. However, in the US healthcare system, we have the resources to actually make it better if we prioritize it.

Destination countries do need to be aware of social accountability and distributive justice. It has been estimated that foreign physician recruitment has saved the US over $846 million in physician education costs alone, while costing countries like South Africa approximately $1.41 billion in lost education costs for physicians who left the country after receiving their education (Mills et al., 2011). It has been noted that for nurses, expenses associated with recruiting abroad, even after including agency fees and foreign nurse integration into the destination country's milieu, are less than educating home-based students (Yeates, 2010).

Consider This

It is within each of us to be globally and ethically accountable to the emigration of nurses. Each nurse, regardless of country of origin, has the freedom to migrate. Many nurses choose to migrate due to poor wages, economic instability, safety issues, poor working conditions, inadequately funded health systems, and political instability (just to name a few). Migration to wealthier countries offers personal resolution to many of these issues. However, source countries are being left with a diminished workforce, populations with decreased access to care, and a drain of the most knowledgeable nurses. This is leading countries to have less access to healthcare resources than high-income countries. Where does our responsibility lie not only for improving the care of our patients in the US, but any human worldwide?

In 2018, 14% of healthcare workers in the US were foreign born (Shaffer et al., 2022). Visa applications rose 109% since 2018 for healthcare workers from 116 countries. In 2022, 81% of new visa applicants were registered nurses (Padilla, 2023). It is important to understand the research and perspectives related to IEN so that a more ethical approach will occur in the future. This information, while limited, should be taken into consideration.

One study concerning problems faced by foreign-educated nurses during 2003–2007 (Pittman et al., 2012) found that 50% of actively recruited foreign-educated nurses experienced a negative recruitment practice. Additionally, the study found that nurses educated in low-income countries and nurses with high contract-breach fees were significantly more likely to report negative experiences (Pittman et al., 2012).

Hospitals and healthcare organizations that utilize foreign-educated nurses need to create action plans around improving communication. Additionally, each of us needs to take an ethical approach and balance between ensuring our own RN workforce from within the US and welcoming migrating nurses.

Tips for healthcare team members working with IENs:

- Be patient and accommodating. Remember that a newly arrived IEN is going through a lot of challenges both at and outside of work. Consider learning about their culture to better understand them.

- Be aware that the care systems where the IENs came from are different from those in the US.

- Create a culturally sensitive educational program for IENs transitioning to practice in your organization with a focus on strengthening their patient safety competencies that are important for maintaining or creating a healthy working environment (HWE)—which can improve nursing retention, a sense of inclusion, satisfaction, and improved patient outcomes.

- Use your diversity, equity, and inclusion (DEI) lens when analyzing situations and resolving concerns. Be open-minded.

- Is the community ready for diversity? Are there resources in your community for the individuals to welcome them to the community, including country- and nation-specific clubs or groups that allow EINs to connect?

Tips for preceptors, educators/NPDS, and nurse leaders (Padilla, 2023):

- Assess the potential knowledge gaps of IENs.

- Set practical expectations with the IEN early in the orientation process.

- Set up consistent, meaningful meetings to check their progress.

- Provide support structures such as a mentorship program.

- Do not consider an IEN's difficulties as incompetence, but rather consider them as a learning opportunity.

- Be aware of their potential challenges and how that may affect their work.

Travel/Registry Nurses

Much like the ebb and flow around foreign nurse recruitment, there are patterns to increased use of travel or registry nurses, peaking during severe shortages. Between 2001 and 2006, usage of supplemental nurses went from 56% of US hospitals to 75% (Xue et al., 2012). Understanding that poor nurse staffing has implications for patient outcomes, registry and travel nurses do have a place in hospital or healthcare organization workforce planning. There are differences between travel RNs and registry RNs (also known as *supplemental RNs*). However, differing from a hospital's internal float RN staff, these RNs are employed by a third party and contract to provide anywhere from one 12-hour shift of service to extended service of six weeks or longer.

Staff RNs and managers have long been concerned with usage of external nurses for fear of decreased quality. Initial research noted higher mortality rates with higher use of supplemental nurses (Aiken et al., 2007); however, when controlling for the quality of the work environment, the association disappeared (Aiken et al., 2013). Fast forward to 2023, adverse associations between travel nursing and patient care may reflect staffing levels or work environments rather than the travel nurses themselves (Vander Weerdt et al., 2023).

Location, Location, Location!

As you have learned, you have many care delivery models to consider, each with a unique impact on your staffing and scheduling. An additional consideration for your care delivery model, productivity, and staffing is the geography of your unit. What is the shape of your unit—racetrack, corridor, or radial? How does each of these floor shapes impact your model and productivity? If you have a corridor-shaped unit, can you have an efficient functional nursing care model? Or if you have a radial-shaped unit, how can you deliver care efficiently in a team-based approach? Again, how do you develop a care delivery model and staff for it in a way that leads to quality patient care? Hendrich and colleagues (2008) note that although no consistent, statistically significant relationship has been found between the various architectural types and nursing time spent with patients, it does impact the distance they travel in a shift.

As noted in the same study by Hendrich et al. (2008), individual nurses across all study units travel between one and five miles per 10-hour daytime shift, and nurses walk less distance during nighttime shifts when most activities and patient tasks decrease. On night shifts, the average distance traveled ranges between 1.3 and 3.3 miles per 10 hours (Hendrich et al., 2008). If you were the nurse who walked one mile, you might be more productive than and not as tired as the nurse who walked five miles in a shift. You might be able to contribute some variation in distance walked to the nurse's aptitude to plan well, but regardless, it is something you must consider and help correct. Although you might not notice walking variations impacting your productivity numbers, you might notice it in nurse fatigue and burnout.

In addition to shape of the unit, other design elements can improve your staff's efficiency and the unit's productivity:

- Single-patient rooms (tend to be larger than double, and more procedures can be done in-room)

- Visible handwashing sinks in each room

- Gel dispensers in all general and patient care areas (every 20–40 feet)

- Computers at the bedside or right outside the room

- Enough computers for everyone to document immediately

- Decentralized nurses' stations (not just one)

- Multiple supply closets, and dirty and clean utilities (not just one positioned in a central location)

- Multiple medications-administration dispensing machines or cubicles (not just one located in a central area)

The shape and layout of your unit do have an impact on how your staff members function and their efficiency and effectiveness in meeting patient needs. Walk your unit and take notes on how your unit may impede or assist your staff.

Summary

Here are the key points covered in this chapter:

- Understanding and standardizing your care delivery model has a major impact on your staffing.

- There are multiple care delivery models, including team-based, modular, primary, and functional.

- Staffing your unit should be in harmony with your care delivery model.

- Have one consistent care delivery model each shift, each day.

- Float teams can offer another level of support.

- Rapid response teams assist in providing another level of support to your unit and help you maximize the scheduling of your novice staff.

- There is an ethical need to balance support for foreign nurse immigration and social accountability.

- Supplemental RN utilization within a good nursing work environment has no significant negative impact on patient outcomes.

- The layout of your unit can impact your staff's efficiency and fatigue level.

References

Aiken, L. H., Sloane, D. M., Bruyneel, L., Van den Heede, K., & Sermeus, W. (2013). Nurses' reports of working conditions and hospital quality of care in 12 countries in Europe. *International Journal of Nursing Studies, 50,* 43–153. https://doi.org/10.1016/j.ijnurstu.2012.11.009

Aiken, L. H., Xue, Y., Clarke, S. P., & Sloane, D. M. (2007). Supplemental nurse staffing in hospitals and quality of care. *Journal of Nursing Administration, 37*(7), 335–342. https://doi.org/10.1097/01.nna.0000285119.53066.ae

Beckett, C. D., Zadvinskis, I. M., Dean, J., Iseler, J., Powell, J. M., & Buck-Maxwell, B. (2021). An integrative review of team nursing and delegation: Implications for nurse staffing during COVID-19. *Worldviews on Evidence-Based Nursing, 18*(4), 251–260. https://doi.org/10.1111/wvn.12523

Chen, Q., Gottlieb, L., Liu, D., Tang, S., & Bai, Y. (2020). The nurse outcomes and patient out-comes following the High-Quality Care Project. *International Nursing Review, 67*(3), 362–371. https://doi.org/10.1111/inr.12587

Healthcare Plus Solutions Group. (2023, March). *Models of care insight study.* https://healthcareplussg.com/models-of-care-insight-study-results/

Hendrich, A., Chow, M. P., Skierczynski, B. A., & Lu, Z. (2008). A 36-hospital time and motion study: How do medical surgical nurses spend their time? *The Permanente Journal, 12*(3), 25–34. https://doi.org/10.7812/tpp/08-021

Lalu, G. P. (2023, May 4). DOH: It will take 12 years for PH to solve shortage of nurses, 23 years for doctors. *The Inquirer.* https://newsinfo.inquirer.net/1764748/doh-it-will-take-12-years-for-ph-to-solve-shortage-of-nurses-23-years-for-doctors#ixzz85LcI9cU2

Litvak, E., & Pronovost, P. J. (2010). Rethinking rapid response teams [Commentary]. *Journal of American Medical Association, 304*(12), 1375–1376. https://doi.org/10.1001/jama.2010.1385

Magnusson, C., Allan, H., Horton, K., Johnson, M., Evans, K., & Ball, E. (2017). An analy-sis of delegation styles among newly qualified nurses. *Nursing Standard, 31*(25). https://doi.org/10.7748/ns.2017.e9780

Mills, E. J., Kanters, S., Hagopian, A., Bansback, N., Nachega, J., Alberton, M., Au-Yeung, C. G., Mtambo, A., Bourgeault, I. L., Luboga, S., Hogg, R. S., & Ford, N. (2011). The financial cost of doctors emigrating from sub-Saharan Africa: Human capital analysis. *BMJ, 343*, d7031. https://doi.org/10.1136/bmj.d7031

Padilla, M. (2023, May 1). *Internationally educated nurses' experiences working in the U.S.* American Association of Critical-Care Nurses. www.aacn.org/blog/internationally-educated-nurses-experiences-working-in-the-us

Pittman, P., Herrera, C., Spetz, J., & Davis, C. R. (2012). Immigration and contract problems experienced by foreign educated nurses. *Medical Care Research and Review, 69*(3), 351–365. https://doi.org/10.1177/1077558711432890

Shaffer, F. A., Bakhshi, M., Cook, K., & Álvarez, T. D. (2022). International nurse recruitment beyond the COVID-19 pandemic: Considerations for the nursing workforce leader. *Nurse Leader, 20*(2), 161–167. https://doi.org/10.1016/j.mnl.2021.12.001

Tiedeman, M. E., & Lookinland, S. (2004). Traditional models of care delivery: What have we learned? *The Journal of Nursing Administration, 34*(6), 291–297. https://doi.org/10.1097/00005110-200406000-00008

Tonkikh, O., Zisberg, A., & Shadmi, E. (2020). Association between continuity of nursing care and older adults' hospitalization outcomes: A retrospective observational study. *Journal of Nursing Management, 28*(5), 1062–1069. https://doi.org/10.1111/jonm.13031

Vander Weerdt, C., Peck, J. A., & Porter, T. (2023). Travel nurse and patient outcomes: A sys-tematic review. *Health Care Management Review, 48*(4), 352–362. https://doi.org/10.1097/HMR.0000000000000383

World Health Organization. (2010, May 20). *WHO global code of practice on the international recruitment of health personnel.* https://www.who.int/publications/i/item/wha68.32

World Health Organization. (2022). *WHO global code of practice on the international recruit-ment of health personnel: Fourth round of national reporting.* https://apps.who.int/gb/ebwha/pdf_files/WHA75/A75_14-en.pdf

Xue, Y., Aiken, L. H., Freund, D. A., & Noyes, K. (2012). Quality outcomes of hospital supple-mental nurse staffing. *The Journal of Nursing Administration, 42*(12), 580–585. https://doi.org/10.1097/NNA.0b013e318274b5bc

Yeates, N. (2010). The globalization of nurse migration: Policy issues and responses. *International Labour Review, 149*(4), 423–440. https://doi.org/10.1111/j.1564-913X.2010.00096.x

Yoder-Wise, P. S. (2003). *Leading and managing in nursing* (3rd ed.). Elsevier.

Zhang, Q., Lee, K., Mansor, Z., Ismail, I., Guo, Y., Xiao, Q., & Lim, P. Y. (2024). Effects of rapid response team on patient outcomes: A systematic review. *Heart & Lung, 63,* 51–64.

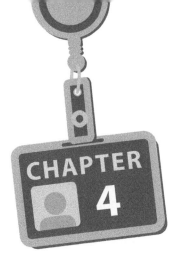

Maximize the Capacity and Capabilities of Your RN Workforce

How many times have you heard someone say, "A nurse is a nurse"? Often this misunderstanding comes from someone in a non–nursing department. Disappointingly, we have also heard this from nursing colleagues. This mentality is then reinforced when we use such calculations as nursing hours per patient day for budget, staffing, and scheduling. It reduces the art and science of nursing into a number, void of context as it treats everyone the same. How do you take into consideration a nurse who has one year of experience compared to one who has 15 years of progressive experience? Can an LPN under the supervision of an RN do everything an RN can do? If someone says, "A nurse is a nurse is a nurse is a nurse is a nurse," that person obviously has never read the legal scope of practice for all nurses.

In this chapter, you will learn how to be innovative with nursing practice through collaboration with stakeholders. Innovation in nursing practice will allow you to think differently about your care delivery model and how you may staff and schedule. Remember, at one point in our nursing history, we were not allowed to use a stethoscope. To successfully innovate, you need to know your professional and specialty organizations' scope and standards of practice as a framework for innovative practice, the self-determination of your staff, state laws and regulations, and professional liability and risk-management concerns, as well as your organization's policies and procedures.

Understanding the Legal Scope of Practice

Have you ever created a schedule where you are happy if you just get all the holes filled? Did you treat an LPN the same as an RN on the schedule? Did you treat the new graduate RN the same as the experienced RN? Have you read the scope of practice for those on your unit, including other disciplines, and taken those factors into consideration? When you are staffing and scheduling your nurses and other personnel, you are setting them up for success or failure in providing quality patient care. To effectively staff and schedule, you must understand all your staff members' legal scope of practice and how their practice may impact your unit's or department's patient productivity and outcomes.

The nursing profession includes many diverse types of licensed nurses: registered nurses (RNs), licensed practical nurses/licensed vocational nurses (LPNs/LVNs), and advanced practice registered nurses (APRNs), which include certified nurse practitioners (CNPs), certified nurse-midwives (CNMs), clinical nurse specialists (CNSs), and certified registered nurse anesthetists (CRNAs). Each type has a legal scope of practice that is governed by the state board of nursing or other type of licensing board in the state where that nurse or APRN holds their license. The legal scope of practice is state-specific and can be slightly different for each type of nurse and APRN. (We review more on APRNs in Chapter 5.) To fully utilize your staff members to their highest current licensed ability, both you and they need to understand their legal scope as defined by your state board of nursing. As you work on innovative practice and staffing, you will need to partner and work with your state board closely.

NOTE

Many states have enacted protected title laws. This means that only RNs or LPNs may call themselves a nurse, and only those who have been legally granted the APRN title can call themselves a CNS, CNP, CNM, or CRNA. This type of law is enacted to protect the public and to stop those who have not been granted these titles from using them. Additionally, some states have passed laws prohibiting APRNs from using the title "Doctor" with any patients. In some states, such misuse may be a felony.

Scope of practice, at minimum, is restricted to what the laws, rules, and regulations in your state permit based on what type of nurse or APRN you are. It is important that you read your scope of practice for the state in which you are licensed and practicing as well as the scope of those you work with and those you staff and schedule. Effective and legal delegation cannot happen unless each licensed individual is aware of their own scope and what can or cannot be delegated to others. You can get to your state's and other states' nursing boards and nurse practice acts through an internet search or via the National Council of State Boards of Nursing website (https://www.ncsbn.org/contactbon.htm).

Consider This

It is important to vote in your state elections! Do not just pay attention to federal races but local ones too. Your elected state legislators have final authority to add, alter, or reduce your scope of practice as an RN or APRN. Go to your state nurses' association website and look for the political action committee (PAC) work. Usually, your state nursing association has vetted candidates for state office based on issues important to nursing as well as candidates understanding of the role nurses play.

Collaborating With Stakeholders on Innovative Practice

Your state's nurse practice act does not cover every act or every scenario that may come up. This can be good and bad. First, let us look at why this could be bad. Reading through the nurse practice act for the appropriate state or states is time consuming. But it's important to understand what is within the professional, educational, and legal scope of an RN, LPN, or APRN so that you can develop innovative or standardized practice guidelines and policies. Making things more complicated, often the legal scope of practice is "silent" on an issue. So, if you are looking for a clear-cut answer on a scope issue, the bad news is you may not find it. In those instances, you may need to email or call the state board of nursing (SBON) with your issue for clarification. In creating policies and innovative practices, work with your SBON to advance practice. Often an organization's risk or legal department places self-imposed limits on staff. This can have a detrimental effect on patient care, innovation, and scope of practice by limiting your ability to fully use your staff. However, just because an organization policy says a nurse or staff can do something does not mean that they can based on their licensed scope of practice.

> **TIP**
>
> *Many state boards have developed opinion papers that discuss their take on whether something is within or out of scope, so be sure to read those to see if they have a perspective on a specific task or intervention. For example, your state's scope-of-practice documentation may be silent on an RN providing mild to moderate anesthesia, but there may be an opinion paper that declares the state board's opinion on the matter.*

Now for the good news: Everything is not defined in the scope of practice; in fact, more is not defined than is. How can that be good? This lack of definition gives you the ability to be innovative with your nurses. So, how do you approach doing something innovative with your staff? With the right process and partnership with your organization and the state board, you might be able to pilot or do an innovative practice!

NOTE

Practice will always evolve positively if practice innovation continues to be driven by nurses.

So, what are the steps to creating innovative nursing practice? Start with the following resources and review the desired innovation with multiple stakeholders (American Nurses Association [ANA], 2012):

- Professional and specialty organizations' scope and standards of practice
- Self-determination
- State laws and regulations
- Professional liability and risk-management concerns
- Organizational policies and procedures

These items are discussed in more detail in the following sections.

Professional and Specialty Organizations' Scope and Standards of Practice

In addition to the ANA's Scope and Standards of Practice, many specialty organizations have a defined scope or position paper on this topic, including:

- American Academy of Nurse Practitioners (AANP)
- American Association of Critical-Care Nurses (AACN)
- American Association of Nurse Anesthesiology (AANA)
- American College of Nurse-Midwives (ACNM)
- American Psychiatric Nurses Association (APNA)
- National Association of Pediatric Nurse Practitioners (NAPNAP)
- Oncology Nursing Society (ONS)
- Society of Pediatric Nurses (SPN), a collaborative effort of the ANA and NAPNAP

These are helpful resources designed to guide decision-making. There are many specialty organizations, and while each focus on the unique scope of their practice, many do collaborate with the ANA and the Nursing Organizations Alliance to address and influence current and emerging nursing practice issues.

> **Consider This**
>
> Note that there is a difference between an innovation and a workaround! Bunpin and colleagues noted that *innovation* is when innovative ideas are adapted, adopted, reconfigured, championed, sponsored, and experienced to help solve or improve healthcare problems, products, or services. *Workarounds* are nonsystematic, temporary approaches to handling work obstacles (2016, p. 122). Workarounds can be a symptom of a system that needs improvements.

Self-Determination

As you think of practicing innovation, think about self-determination. *Self-determination* is when nurses determine whether they can perform an act or intervention safely. This includes consideration of their skills, expertise, the clinical setting, and the skills and expertise of other members of the healthcare team (ANA, 2012). In writing your plan, include these items:

- Define the individual who can perform the act or intervention.

- Describe the education, training, precepting, and evaluation method you will use to determine competence. Do not forget ongoing evaluation.

- Determine in which unit or setting this act or intervention can be performed. Are there units in which this cannot be done?

- Identify whether there is a need to have additional support available during the act or intervention. Describe what that support looks like.

- Determine the desired outcome, how you will measure it, and to whom you will report it.

This information will inform your plan, policy, and procedures as you write them.

State Laws and Regulations

If you have not already, you will need to review your state's laws and regulations (nurse practice act) and opinion papers. Consider the following:

- Does the law or regulation discuss an act or intervention, or is it silent on the potential practice? If the law or regulation speaks to it and allows it, great! You can proceed to the next step.

- If the practice is not allowed, schedule a time to talk or meet with the state-board staff member in charge of practice. Can you work on a pilot to demonstrate outcomes? Is there flexibility to do the innovation a little differently? Bring any research or articles that support the practice as well as a detailed plan on the innovation and why you want to implement it.

State laws and regulations need to be followed at all times. If a law or regulation does not make sense, there are avenues to take to change it. Although that may seem like an impossible task, your state nurses association may be the place to start to look for help.

Professional Liability and Risk-Management Concerns

A crucial step is to learn how your hospital's legal and risk department personnel will react to this innovation. Will they see it as something they do not want the hospital to engage in due to the additional risk it might bring? Unfortunately, many nurse managers do not understand that this department provides support services, so when the folks from the legal and risk department tell them no, they go no further. Here is what you need to consider when working with this department:

- Work with individuals in this department to help them understand operationally why this is important. Often *you* as the nurse are the expert in nursing practice.

- Partner with a key executive who is supportive of this change.

- Approach individuals in this department with the attitude that you are seeking their help to make this innovation workable or palatable to the organization's level of risk-taking.

- Schedule a meeting with all key stakeholders to discuss the change, including the executive who supports it.

- If the first answer is no, continue to collaborate to figure out how to make it a yes.

The legal and risk department has your organization's well-being in mind. Although at times they may seem like barriers, employees in this department are not all clinicians and may need extra assistance and time in understanding your request and needs.

Organizational Policies and Procedures

Many of us work in an environment that has a policy and procedure on everything, which stifles innovation and true evidence-based practice. Does a policy or procedure need to be changed, rewritten, or retired to allow this innovative practice? This is when you may hear those infamous words, "That's not the way we do things here." The important thing about organizational policies is that they are easier to change than state law! Consider this:

- Who is the owner of the policy? Talk with them about the desire to change.

- Did you talk with your boss, and did your boss talk with the chief nurse executive (CNE)? The CNE is usually the individual who signs off on the final copy of the policy and approves all nursing practices. Is there organizational approval to move forward?

No one said being innovative was easy. Nursing practice will need to advance to meet future care delivery models as our healthcare system changes. This will have an impact on how you staff and schedule. The nursing care of your patients tomorrow will be delivered through care delivery models that may not exist today and are waiting for you to develop.

Shared Governance

Shared governance provides the opportunity for staff to be a part of the decision-making process over their practice. This should not be limited to nurses only but all disciplines. For nurses, shared governance activities include participation in research and evidence-based practice projects, as well as determining things such as clinical practices, approving policies and procedures, new equipment, and staffing to name a few. Inclusion will increase by-in, decrease workarounds, and improve staff satisfaction.

Accounting for Competencies, Years of Experience, Education, and Certification

Do you take into consideration the competencies, years of experience, education, and certifications of your nurses and APRNs when you create your schedule? What impact would these factors have on your patient outcomes? You may have several certified oncology nurses one day and only one the next. This may be due to many issues, including the expense in paying for certifications, but how much time do you even spend trying to make the schedule based on these factors?

Consider This

Research has shown that years of nursing experience did not have an impact on patient outcomes (Kendall-Gallagher et al., 2011). Why? In some cases, 20 years of experience means 20 years of building education, certifications, and competencies. In other cases, nurses may have been stagnant, not progressing to a bachelor of science in nursing (BSN), not becoming certified, or not maintaining competencies. In other words, they might have repeated their first year of nursing 20 times. So, do not equate years of experience with competency.

We know that certifications and BSN-prepared nurses lead to better patient outcomes, including lower 30-day mortality and failure-to-rescue rates for surgical patients. Every 10% increase in baccalaureate-prepared nurses with certification has been associated with a 2% decrease in the odds of a patient dying (Kendall-Gallagher et al., 2011). Additionally, in hospitals with more baccalaureate-trained colleagues and lower nurse workloads, nurses have demonstrated a greater opportunity to recognize patient deterioration before cardiac arrest and institute life-saving interventions (Harrison et al., 2019). Further research has found that better outcomes were attributed in large part to highly qualified and educated nurses, including a higher proportion of baccalaureate-prepared RNs (McHugh & Ma, 2013). So why would we not ensure that every nurse could obtain a BSN (or is in school) and is certified? Most importantly, why is it OK for staff to have varying levels of nursing competency, education, and certification shift to shift, day by day, if we know these factors do make a difference in patient care and outcomes?

NOTE

We're not arguing for BSN entry only. But with every degree completed, most nurses learn more to improve not only patient outcomes but systems of outcomes too.

We do not want to make this an argument that one person is better than another or one's skills are better. This is about education level, not the person—BSN versus associate degree or diploma nurses. When an organization such as the Institute of Medicine creates the report *The Future of Nursing: Leading Change, Advancing Health,* in which even physicians argue that 80% of RNs should be BSN-prepared by 2020, it is time to get on board. Support, encourage, and push your staff in completing advanced degrees and certifications. As of 2022, over 70% of RNs had a bachelor's degree or higher (Smiley et al., 2023).

Student Nurses

So, you have created this great schedule (or you think you have), and along comes an administrator or faculty member of a nursing school wanting to place students on your unit. What are you thinking? We hope you are the type of manager who is excited to be involved in preparing for the future generation of nurses.

Just as we need to be innovative with our staff, we can partner on being innovative with nursing students. They need clinical experience, and you have a ton of duties that need to get done that are clinical in nature! Do not think of students as a drain on your resources but as an extra free resource (who need experience). You may be wondering how a nursing student can help your staffing and productivity. First, you should change your mindset. Here is one example of innovation with nursing students.

Creative Partnership Between Staff and Students

Hospitals traditionally provide a wonderful proving ground for training in assessment, time management, teamwork, and care planning. Finding an opportunity to teach nursing students that would not tax nursing load while ensuring value gave rise to a creative solution. The model that was utilized to provide an excellent learning experience supported staffing a required, quarterly, house-wide patient assessment. As part of the National Database of Nursing Quality Indicators, patient-safety assessments (particularly for pressure ulcer prevalence and incidence) require significant labor to perform effectively.

To staff this, we initially sought staff who could be removed from the bedside. This proved to be a daunting request, especially during high-volume, high-acuity cycles. We proposed to have a nursing student accompany a trained survey nurse to assist with the study. The student was able to facilitate positioning and patient care as needed while appreciating observational teaching moments, including a skin assessment and prevention and intervention measures.

Upon completion of the day, each student had encountered and observed an average of 60 patient assessments. This not only increased the students' exposure to the serious process of monitoring patient safety and outcomes but also minimized the impact on staffing and reduced the number of staff needed to complete the study.

–Judy L. Gates, MSN, RN, BC, CWS, FACCWS

How do you find those innovative partnerships with your unit and the nursing students? If your organization has someone who coordinates the nursing colleges and students, connect with them first. Then do the following:

1. Find out what each semester's nursing students need for experiences.

2. Plan: Look at your unit's needs and match them with experiences for specific semesters.

3. Talk with your contacts at the nursing school. Chances are, what you need help with will not account for an entire clinical rotation, but it may give a great clinical experience for a day or two that also helps with your unit's workload.

Remember, nursing students practice under the license of their instructor and their nurse preceptor. They do not have a scope of practice because they are not licensed. The nursing school will collaborate with you to ensure the students do not go beyond their student scope.

New Graduate RNs

We move from a free resource for your unit, the nursing student, to the costliest and most resource-intensive, the new graduate RN. (*New graduate RNs* are typically defined as those within their first 12 months post-licensure.) Talk about implications for your schedule and staffing! Outside of scheduling their orientation to your unit and those first several months, continuing to collaborate with new graduates through the first year is important. After they have "graduated" from their orientation and no longer have a preceptor helping them care for patients, we frequently add them to the schedule as if they were equal to any other nurse.

The National Council of State Boards of Nursing (NCSBN, 2012) and the state boards of nursing noted that over the years, there have been many issues with the training and retention of new nurses. One key finding is the inability of new nurses to properly transition into practice, which can have grave consequences (NCSBN, 2012):

- New nurses care for sicker patients in increasingly complex health settings.

- More than 40% of new nurses report making medication errors.

- New nurses feel increased stress levels, which is a risk factor for patient safety and practice errors.

- Approximately 25% of new nurses leave a position within their first year of practice.

- Increased turnover negatively influences patient safety and healthcare outcomes.

Since before the COVID-19 pandemic, the United States has faced a nursing shortage. As usual, schools have increased production of RNs, and hospitals have hired increasingly larger numbers of new graduate RNs. Onboarding large numbers of new graduate nurses leads to higher rates of preceptor burnout, higher turnover of new graduate nurses in their first year of employment, and higher staffing costs with no improvement in outcomes. To address this issue, some hospitals have opened what has been termed a *new graduate unit*, *designated transition unit*, or *nursing education training unit*. While that may not be a new idea, it is an idea that continues to come and go as a solution to first-year turnover and the heavy needs of orienting new graduate nurses.

Here are some points to consider when staffing and scheduling new graduates:

- Have they completed all competencies needed to work unrestricted on the unit?

- Should their productivity be the same as a nurse who is not a new graduate? Consider extended periods of scheduling once off orientation that does not expect the same productivity as an experienced nurse.

- Do you start new graduate RNs with a patient load the same as more experienced RNs, or do you gradually increase their workload as they gain experience over many months?

- Do you expect your other nurses to pick up the differences in productivity to meet your budget of FTEs and hours per patient day?

- Do you work with your finance department and boss to assign a different weight to your new graduates as partial productive FTEs?

- Do you work with your charge nurses or staff to ensure the gradual increase in productivity over the first year?

See Chapter 9 for more on innovative transition units.

Experienced RNs

Experienced RNs make up less and less of the direct care acute care workforce. One area of focus for the experienced RN has been what the literature calls the *aging workforce* and *wisdom at work*, which, post-COVID-19, has never been more important.

> **Consider This**
>
> The term *aging workforce* is often wrongly used to mean experienced or expert nurses. It implies in some sense that older nurses must be experts or have many years of experience behind them. Do not automatically assume the 60-year-old nurses have 40 years of experience. They may have the same 20 years of experience as the 40-year-olds!

The terms *aging workforce* and *wisdom at work* are not synonymous, but they are related. The aging workforce refers to those nurses who are older and may be approaching retirement in 10 to 15 years. Wisdom at work relates to keeping experienced nurses in the work setting rather than losing their knowledge, which must be relearned by younger, less-experienced nurses, with resulting impacts on cost and organizational performance (Robert Wood Johnson Foundation [RWJF], 2010). Many organizations have attempted various methods to retain these nurses. In a study supported by the RWJF from 2006 to 2010, of the

13 initiatives aimed at retaining experienced nurses, four were considered staffing projects and are even more relevant today (RWJF, 2010):

- **Using closed staffing as a nursing retention strategy:** A nurse staffing model that keeps nurses on their home units rather than assigning them to other units as needed.

- **Specialized admission role to ease patient gridlock and help retain experienced nurses:** A program relying on specially designated and experienced admission nurses to facilitate patient admission.

- **Impact of the base staffing model on retention of experienced nurses:** A nurse staffing model that staffs for frequent peak occupancy rather than average occupancy.

- **Giving experienced nurses more control over patient flow, discharge, and admission:** A program that uses experienced nurses to manage patient admission and placement

Results of these initiatives varied; however, case studies of the top-performing organizations reported that successful retention of experienced nurses focused on two factors (RWJF, 2010):

1. Corporate culture of valuing experienced workers

2. Structured, organization-wide focus on management and developing talent

If you have an aging workforce, these are initiatives to try on your unit or in your organization.

LPNs/LVNs

LPNs/LVNs are nurses who practice under the supervision of the registered nurse or physician. (There is typically no difference in practice between an LPN and an LVN, just the state's preference in naming convention.) Just like the RN, the LPN has a scope of practice defined by each state board outlining their role and functions within the license. The LPN educational requirement can vary from state to state but is approximately one year and can be obtained at a vocational school or community college. Although LPNs can practice in a hospital setting, the long-term care setting has been a significant place of employment. Post-COVID-19, as the RN shortage worsens, more hospitals are looking at the team model of care, which means looking to hire more LPNs. (Chapter 3 introduces the different models of care.)

When hired into the acute care setting, LPNs are usually part of a team-based nursing care delivery model on a medical-surgical unit, where patient acuity is less than in a progressive or intensive care setting. In a team-based approach, the RN delegates interventions and tasks to the LPN, and the LPN documents and reports back to the RN as the team lead. A key point to successful incorporation of LPNs within the acute care setting is to minimize role confusion by being consistent with role responsibilities (Alexander, 2022).

NOTE

When an LPN is working with an RN, they are collaborating with the delegation of that RN, so RNs may be afraid of losing their license if the LPN does something wrong. It is important to emphasize to RNs and LPNs that each license has its own legal scope of practice. If LPNs do something that violates their own scope through their own actions (not from inappropriate delegation but by acting independently), they will be held accountable for their own actions. RNs may be held accountable if they delegate something to LPNs that is beyond their scope or competency.

There are many benefits to using an LPN on the team, particularly reduced costs in staffing. Remember, the research has shown that the more RN hours per patient, the better the outcomes (Kane et al., 2007). Keep in mind the cost of adverse events and hospital-acquired conditions. These costs may outweigh the savings of not going to an RN-only nurse model. These costs and benefits will need to be reviewed at your unit level to determine what is best for your patients. (Further benefits and potential issues of team-based nursing are reviewed in Chapter 3.)

Here are some things to consider when staffing and scheduling an LPN:

- They need to understand their scope of practice.
- If they can do additional tasks with certification (e.g., IVs), ensure there is a certificate on file, and it is current.
- Ensure the RNs scheduled at the same time understand the scope of practice for the LPN.
- Make sure the RNs scheduled at the same time feel comfortable with and are knowledgeable about appropriate delegation.
- Be sure the LPN understands the chain of command and takes direction from the RN for all aspects of the nursing process.
- Do not schedule the LPN with higher numbers of novice or newer RNs.

Depending on your care delivery model, LPNs can be additional resources for your team. Ensure that your RNs are knowledgeable in delegation principles and know their role with LPNs.

NAPs

NAP (nursing assistive personnel) is the updated language for what had been called UAPs, or unlicensed assistive personnel, and are used in many areas across the acute care setting. Typically, NAPs consist of nursing assistants, sitters, patient care assistants, and other non-licensed healthcare providers; however, they may hold certifications. NAPs should always work under the direction of an RN, LPN, or other licensed professional. NAPs do have some formal or on-the-job training. The use of these individuals may be part of a primary nursing model (the sole support of the RN) or part of a team-based approach. NAPs do save a unit money and assist the nurse in completing tasks or interventions that can be delegated and do not require a license to perform.

NOTE

What is the difference between a nursing assistant and certified nursing assistant (CNA)? CNAs attended an approved school (regulations governed by the Centers for Medicare & Medicaid Services [CMS]) and successfully passed their certifying exam. Nursing assistants do not have a certification and may have been educated through on-the-job training. Different hospitals may call nursing assistants different names, including patient care technicians. CNAs have a scope and fall under some type of state regulation, the state board of nursing. CMS regulations require nursing assistants to be certified in nursing homes and home healthcare. Nursing assistants do not fall under the scope of the state board of nursing.

Sitters are NAPs who "sit" with patients who may be confused, at risk for falls, or on suicide precautions. Sitters may or may not perform nursing-assistant functions while at the patient's bedside, depending on whether your unit or organization has chosen to orient and determine their competency in providing that level of care. Typically, sitters do minimal direct care with these patients. Sitters may be an additional cost to your unit, unlike other NAPs. Because you cannot predict the need for sitters, they may cause you to exceed the budget for your care delivery model. However, the overall organization may save money to offset costs for reductions in falls.

Consider This

If you are considering or have a sitter program, look at the cost/benefit of training the sitters as nursing assistants. It is an additional cost to have an individual sitting at the bedside who cannot perform basic personal-care tasks, such as bathing and turning. Remember: Based on your organizational policies and principles of delegation, an RN cannot delegate a task to anyone unless they know that person received the proper training and is competent to perform that task—even a task as simple as a bed bath or ambulating the patient to the bathroom.

For evaluation of benefits over potential issues of the use of NAPs in your care delivery model, review Chapter 3 and the various nursing care delivery models.

Health Unit Clerks/Ward Secretaries

Unit clerks, health secretaries, or ward secretaries serve a vital role in a paper or hybrid medical record world. They also are the face of your unit, greeting patients, family, and physicians. Traditionally, this role has impacted the nurses positively by decreasing the paperwork burden through taking off orders, calling in orders, and facilitating the flow of patients. But as practices and regulations have changed, so has their role. Many nurse managers have found that as they transition to an electronic health record (EHR), including computerized provider order entry, the role of the unit secretary has changed. As this role is re-envisioned or reconsidered, think about the workflow of your unit or department and what can be taken off nurses' to-do lists that does not require a license to do. To allow nurses to practice to the highest degree of their license, non-licensed-required functions will need to be delegated to others.

As you implement an EHR, here are some points to consider for your unit clerk staffing:

- Do you need a unit clerk on every shift?

- Do you need a unit clerk only during certain high-call-volume times?

- What other tasks completed by the unit clerk might be made automatic?

- Are there tasks not getting done that can be delegated to this individual?

- Can you share a unit clerk across multiple units instead of having one for each unit?

As technology changes, the role of the unit clerk has evolved. As you look for efficiency in your budget and staffing, this may be one area of opportunity.

Summary

Here are the key points covered in this chapter:

- A nurse is not a nurse is not a nurse; hours per patient day and other metrics strip the context of nursing practice.

- All licensed nurses have a scope of practice; read them all.

- Recognize the difference between an innovation and a workaround.

- To create innovative nursing practice, you will need to collaborate with a whole host of stakeholders.

- Innovation and change do not come easily. Someone might tell you no the first time you ask to change a practice that has always been the way your organization does it.

- Understand the nursing players on your unit, their scopes, and their abilities so you can maximize your staffing.

References

Alexander, M. (2022). Maximizing the role of the LPN. *Journal of Nursing Regulation, 13*(1), 3. https://doi.org/10.1016/S2155-8256(22)00027-8

American Nurses Association. (2012). *Nurse staffing plans & ratios*. http://www.nursingworld. org/MainMenuCategories/Policy-Advocacy/State/Legislative-Agenda-Reports/State-Staffing-PlansRatios/default.aspx

Bunpin, J. J., Chapman, S., Blegan, M., & Spetz, J. (2016). Differences in innovative behavior among hospital based registered nurses. *The Journal of Nursing Administration, 46*(3), 122–127. https://doi.org/10.1097/NNA.0000000000000310

Harrison, J. M., Aiken, L. H., Sloane, D. M., Brooks Carthon, J. M., Merchant, R. M., Berg, R. A., & McHugh, M. D. (2019). In hospitals with more nurses who have baccalaureate degrees, better outcomes for patients after cardiac arrest. *Health Affairs, 38*(7), 1087–1094. https://doi.org/10.1377/hlthaff.2018.05064

Kane, R. L., Shamliyan, T. A., Mueller, C., Duval, S., & Wilt, T. J. (2007). The association of registered nurse staffing levels and patient outcomes: Systematic review and meta-analysis. *Medical Care, 45*(12), 1195–1204. https://doi.org/10.1097/MLR.0b013e3181468ca3

Kendall-Gallagher, D., Aiken, L. H., Sloane, D. M., & Cimiotti, J. P. (2011). Nurse specialty certification, inpatient mortality, and failure to rescue. *Journal of Nursing Scholarship, 43*, 188–194. https://doi.org/10.1111/j.1547-5069.2011.01391.x

McHugh, M. D, & Ma, C. (2013). Hospital nursing and 30-day readmissions among Medicare patients with heart failure, acute myocardial infarction, and pneumonia. *Medical Care, 51*(1), 52–59. https://doi.org/10.1097/MLR.0b013e3182763284

National Council of State Boards of Nursing. (2012). *Transition to practice.* https://www.ncsbn.org/nursing-regulation/practice/transition-to-practice.page

Robert Wood Johnson Foundation. (2010). *Wisdom at work: Retaining experienced nurses: An RWJF national program.* http://rwjf.org/files/research/WWN.final.pdf

Smiley, R. A., Allgeyer, R. L., Shobo, Y., Lyons, K. C., Letourneau, R., Zhong, E., Kaminski-Ozturk, N., & Alexander, M. (2023). The 2022 National Nursing Workforce Survey. *Journal of Nursing Regulation, 14*(1), S1–S90. https://doi.org/10.1016/S2155-8256(23)00047-9

Empower All Disciplines to Practice to Their Full Scope

We have all heard at some point that only an RN can do something. Sometimes, it is true. Oftentimes it is the nurses who want to keep doing tasks that are delegable, such as starting IVs. As a leader and innovator for care delivery models, we need to figure out what the rest of our healthcare team can and does do every day based on their scopes of practice. Although the focus is mainly on nurse staffing in this book, consider the other disciplines on the team as you look at staffing, scheduling, or your care delivery model. Care delivery does not happen with nurses only; nurses and patients rely on a team of educated healthcare professionals to help deliver that care. Depending on your model, a physician or nurse may lead the care. Models that use the most appropriate disciplines, with the RN as the care coordinator, are promising models for tomorrow.

To be as effective as possible in providing care, we must be *interprofessional*—professionals who learn with, from, and about each other to improve collaboration and quality of care. In this chapter, we will look at the other essential healthcare team members, their practice, and how they can impact staffing.

Assessing the Impact of All Staff and Disciplines on Patient Care

Understanding the role and scope of other disciplines in the hospital and on your unit is essential. This understanding will continue to drive the evolution of your care delivery model and clarify who might be best for which task. For example, the clinical nurse specialist (CNS) is used frequently in a nurse educator role on a unit instead of taking advantage of their full scope of advanced practice licensed. Nurses often are assigned medication reconciliation, but what if a pharmacist or pharmacy technician performed this role instead? Do you have RN and medical social workers who act as case managers who focus on medical and social aspects of discharge planning? Would that free up time for the direct care nurses to do other things? Understanding the roles of other disciplines gives you insight into who can do the work and how it can be redesigned to be more efficient and effective to really create the care delivery models we need today.

 NOTE

Many more individuals—such as physician assistants; physical, occupational, or speech therapists; and dietitians—impact the team, but this chapter does not cover them. However, they are just as crucial to your care delivery model, so make sure you also know their roles, scopes of practice, and the research that demonstrates their unique contribution to patient care.

Working With Stakeholders on Innovative Practice

When it comes to innovation in practice for APRNs and others, use the same process of stakeholder collaboration as noted in Chapter 4. The difference may be driven based on whether your state has a regulatory agency or board that governs the profession. As is true for nursing, there are variations in practice state to state for many other disciplines. Become familiar with your state's practice acts and regulations for all healthcare disciplines.

Some states may not be clear in scope. For instance, Alaska has no board for respiratory therapists (RTs), thus no license for RTs. However, Alaska does require that RTs graduate from a nationally accredited RT program. The question for RTs in that state is: Who determines practice, and who should be at the table when discussing practice innovation? In the following sections of this chapter, we discuss other disciplines and their roles and give examples of their actual and potential impact on the unit.

Advanced Practice Registered Nurses

To decrease the variation for advance practice registered nurses (APRNs), the APRN Consensus Model convened a group of stakeholders to agree upon license, accreditation, certification, and education (LACE) requirements for each APRN role. While the original document was published in 2008, as of 2023, there was a group reconvened to determine updates to this model that are not currently published. The APRN Consensus Model for Regulation (2008) designates four advanced practice registered nurse (APRN) roles:

- Certified nurse practitioner (CNP)
- Clinical nurse specialist (CNS)
- Certified nurse-midwife (CNM)
- Certified registered nurse anesthetist (CRNA)

Each role will impact your staffing and scheduling, whether your unit or organization employs these individuals, or these individuals have an independent practice in your organization. It cannot be said enough that often organizational policies and antiquated medical staff rules artificially limit an APRN's practice, even in a state with independent or full practice authority. These violations of free trade need to end, and the Federal Trade Commission (FTC) has proposed that state policymakers enable APRNs and physician assistants (PAs) to be fully authorized to practice in accordance with their education, training, and experience (2014).

NOTE

The primary issue with practice innovation with APRNs is that the hospital's Medical Staff Committee needs to allow them to function to the extent they are licensed independently. Many blame the hospital for restricting APRN practice. It is important to understand that the Medical Staff Committee, which oversees quality at the hospital and governs itself (granted and regulated through the Centers for Medicare & Medicaid Services, or CMS), is a separate entity from the hospital. Hospital administration personnel cannot tell the medical staff they must do something; however, they can work with committee members to progress their thinking on this and many other important topics.

Many staffing and scheduling tools need to consider these APRN roles as individuals (as employees). Consider the impact on your scheduling and staffing with these individuals if they were your employees. What type of care model improvements could be made to your unit or department? Suppose these individuals round on your unit as non-employed medical staff members. In that case, they still impact your unit's flow and how you schedule, such as improving discharge timeliness, addressing patient and clinician questions more quickly, and attending rounds that should facilitate and collaborate with the team on the patient's care plan toward their discharge. (This will be discussed more in Chapter 6.)

NOTE

Looking at the titles, you may think, "I have never seen a CNP," or, "That's not what our organization calls them." Do not worry; they are NPs. With the overall title of CNP, state licensing bodies may have different regulations on the exact way an NP must note their credentials.

Certified Nurse Practitioners

According to the APRN Consensus Model for Regulation (2008), the certified nurse practitioner (CNP), or nurse practitioner (NP), provides care along the wellness-illness continuum through a dynamic process in primary and acute care settings. CNPs are prepared to practice as primary care CNPs and acute care CNPs, which have separate national consensus-based competencies and certification processes (APRN, 2008).

Numerous studies have noted the effectiveness of CNPs. The earliest study on the cost and effectiveness of nurse practitioners, completed in 1981 by the Office of Technology Assessment (OTA), reported that NPs provided equivalent or improved medical care at a lower cost than physicians. Many studies have found nurse practitioners provide care with similar outcomes with decreased utilization (Liu et al., 2020). Additionally, a systematic review of 37 studies found consistent evidence that cost-related outcomes such as length of stay, emergency visits, and hospitalizations for NP care are equivalent to those of physicians (Newhouse et al., 2011). A survey in *CHEST* journal found that staffing models that included daytime use of CNPs were safe and effective alternatives to a traditional house staff–based team in a high-acuity adult ICU (Gersherngorn et al., 2011).

Each CNP does the following (APRN, 2008):

- Provides initial, ongoing, and comprehensive care, including taking comprehensive histories, providing physical examinations and other health-assessment and screening activities, and diagnosing, treating, and managing patients with acute and chronic illnesses and diseases

- Orders, performs, supervises, and interprets laboratory and imaging studies; prescribes medication and durable medical equipment; and makes appropriate referrals for patients and families

Use of a Dual-Certificate APRN on a Cardiac ICU Unit

Our APRN has a dual degree as an APRN serving as a CNS and acute care nurse practitioner (ACNP). The combination of both degrees has been influential in advancing nurses' knowledge. To accomplish this, Jennifer collaborates with nurses and physicians to develop order sets and protocols while continually focusing on process improvement and medical management. The dual background has successfully established the Extracorporeal Membrane Oxygenation (ECMO) program, wherein she used her skills to collaborate with critical care nurses, surgeons, and hospital intensivists from the beginning.

Jennifer conducts monthly process-improvement meetings about the program, resulting in process changes. She is dedicated to continuing education and conducts quarterly education and simulation for nurses and physicians to improve the program with positive patient outcomes in extremely critically ill patients.

–Dana Lauer, MS, RN, NEA-BC

It has also been found that having more NPs in hospitals has favorable effects on patients, staff nurse satisfaction, and efficiency, even taking into account favorable nurse to patient ratios (Aiken et al., 2021). Additionally, this enhanced model of care achieved better outcomes with lower spending per episode of care (Aiken et al., 2021). Here is the potential impact of CNPs on staffing:

- Decrease your staff's need to call and wait for orders to change or progress care, leading to efficient nursing care and shorter lengths of stay

- Spend more time at the patient's bedside, leading to improved patient satisfaction and outcomes and decreasing staff time in finding the physician to talk with the patient

- Spend more time in the moment educating your staff, building a more confident and competent staff (part of a CNP's core competency is to continue to develop nursing science and educate others)

- Round at the right time to facilitate improvement in length of stay and discharge, which can help you better manage staffing levels and fluctuations in staffing needs

Consider This

Nurse practitioners in an inpatient setting typically follow industry physician productivity standards even if employed and paid with a salary. The measurement is called Relative Value Units (RVUs). Medicare pays for services based on the submission of a claim using one or more specific Current Procedural Terminology (CPT) codes. CPT codes are numbers assigned to every task and service a medical practitioner may provide to a patient, including medical, surgical, and diagnostic services. Each CPT code has an RVU assigned to it, which, when multiplied by the conversion factor (CF) and a geographical adjustment (GPCI), creates the compensation level for a particular service.

Your hospital may have determined the number of RVUs needed to meet set productivity standards for employed physicians and CNPs. These productivity standards can help you determine how many CNPs you may need on your unit and provide a comparison for benchmarking to other units or organizations. Other CNP productivity measures could include visits or dollars/revenue.

The CNP is a valuable member of the care team as a provider. Work with your organization and CNPs to remove barriers that prohibit them from their full scope of practice. With their full scope and ability, the CNP will be able to provide quality, cost-effective care to your patients and be an excellent mentor for your staff. The Balanced Budget Act of 1997 granted NPs the ability to directly bill Medicare for services that they perform. However, reimbursement is only provided at 85% of the physician rate. However, much work continues to advocate for full payment parity at the federal level.

Several states have considered legislation for pay parity for NPs: however, this impacts only private insurances. Oregon was the first state in the nation to require insurance companies to follow "equal pay for equal work" rules on insurance reimbursements for nurse practitioners, physician assistants, and physicians in primary care and mental health.

Clinical Nurse Specialists

A clinical nurse specialist (CNS) is an advanced practice registered nurse with graduate preparation from a program that prepares CNSs. A CNS and a CNP are not interchangeable; they have different educational preparations and certification tests. The CNS's role is to integrate care across the continuum and through three spheres of influence: patient, nurse, and system (APRN, 2008).

The critical elements of CNS practice are to create environments through mentoring and system changes that empower nurses to develop caring, evidence-based practices (EBPs) to alleviate patient distress, facilitate ethical decision-making, and respond to diversity (APRN, 2008). CNSs are clinical experts in a specialized area. They are responsible and accountable for the diagnosis and treatment of health/illness states, disease management, health promotion, and prevention of illness and risk behaviors among individuals, families, groups, and communities (APRN, 2008).

Numerous studies have documented the impact of the CNS in preventing hospital-acquired conditions (HACs) in acute care settings, usually through CNS-led initiatives. A recent systematic review concluded that utilizing CNSs in a hospital setting reduced the length of stay and decreased care costs while improving patient outcomes (Newhouse et al., 2011). A study published in 2022 noted that a CNS-led program demonstrated reductions in device utilization and catheter infection rates (Pajerski et al., 2022). Another study by Hays (2010) noted that CNSs decreased the HAC rate by 46% in an acute care setting. Additionally, a pressure ulcer treatment program implemented by a CNS decreased HAC rates from 20% to 3.8%, resulting in a cost saving of more than $40,000 for that organization (Richardson & Tjoelker, 2012). Richardson and Tjoelker (2012) also noted that a CNS-led initiative to decrease central line-associated bloodstream infections (CLABSI) saved the organization $214,712 in cost avoidance and 1.4 lives out of 8 patients with CLABSI.

The "Impact of a CNS on Women and Infant Services" sidebar explains how a CNS significantly reduced the C-section rate in one medical center. How would you staff differently if your C-section rate dropped from 20% to 10%, or your OB patients' labor time was significantly reduced? CNSs can have a tangible impact on your patients, impacting your staffing.

Here is the potential impact of CNSs on staffing:

- Develop new innovative nursing care methods that improve patient care

- Continuously educate your staff, leading to a more competent workforce

- Improve engagement of your staff nurses, leading to less turnover

- Provide direct patient care with potential to prescribe medications

Impact of a CNS on Women and Infant Services

Our CNS is a consultant to assist the bedside RN in resolving complex patient-care issues and provides as-needed "hands-on" assistance with nursing care tasks. The CNS has the unique opportunity to support and mentor the RN at the bedside, which aids in their time management and productivity.

Our CNS's focus on EBP and research has engaged and energized the staff. For example, our Newborn Congenital Heart Disease Pulse Oximetry Screening Program was developed by our CNS through collaboration with unit management and bedside RNs. Outcomes of this collaborative approach included the development of engaged bedside champions, joint identification of educational needs, financial analysis review, examination/resolution of bedside RN concerns, consideration of the impact on nursing time, analysis of patient safety factors, and creation of data evaluation tools. Using this leadership model by the CNS provided RN mentorship in teamwork and innovative program development. It provided staff members at the bedside with the ability to see how they could make a difference in patient care.

Our CNS's leadership on a project with a significant quality outcome began with a labor and delivery (L&D) RN's observation of the apparent effect of using a peanut ball on labor. (A *peanut ball* is an exercise ball shaped like a peanut.) Women with epidurals cannot hold their legs apart on their own, which is needed to open the pelvis and birthing canal. Placing a peanut ball between a laboring woman's legs facilitates opening the birthing canal and is thought to aid a natural delivery. Our CNS developed it into an institutional review board (IRB)-approved randomized control study, with bedside L&D RNs participating in the study design and data collection. The study demonstrated significant results of a shortened length of labor, decreased use of vacuum and forceps, and reduction in cesarean sections in labor patients with an epidural. It went on to win our system's highest team-performance excellence award. This research continued its impact as a best practice when rolled out system-wide to our sister hospitals. This outcome highlights how a collaborative partnership between a CNS and bedside nurses can improve the quality of care and advance nursing practice.

Finally, because professional certification is associated with better patient outcomes, our CNS is committed to promoting and supporting professional staff development. Over time, her influence has resulted in our department proudly having 114 certified RNs.

–Carol Olson, MBA, BSN, RN

As primary care practitioners, CNSs can also be reimbursed by Medicare, billing for their services using CPT evaluation and management codes like CNPs. Reimbursement may help with any financial proforma needed to demonstrate the cost/benefit of adding a CNS. However, not all CNS activities result in a CPT code.

NOTE

The National Association of Clinical Nurse Specialists (NACNS) provides many wonderful resources on their website (https://nacns.org), including a sample job description including all the domains of a CNS and a cost analysis tool to help support clinical best practice, among other useful resources.

Therefore, defining productivity standards for CNSs is more challenging, making it harder for you to quantify your needs for CNSs in your unit's staffing and scheduling. Staffing for CNSs on your unit will be based on your patient population and the needs of your staff RNs in combination with your budget. CNSs, when allowed to practice to their full licensure and scope, can positively impact your nurses, patients, and care delivery model.

Certified Nurse-Midwives

According to the APRN Consensus Model (2008), a certified nurse-midwife (CNM) provides a full range of primary healthcare services to women throughout the life span, including gynecological care, family planning services, preconception care, prenatal and postpartum care, childbirth, and care of the newborn. In 2019, 89% of CNMs attended births in the hospital, and unlike CNPs, CNMS are paid at 100% of physician rates for Medicare or Medicaid (American College of Nurse-Midwives, 2019). *The Lancet* (2014) noted that midwifery plays a crucial role in saving the lives of millions of women and children during and around the time of pregnancy. International experts note the scale of the positive impact that can be achieved when effective, high-quality midwifery is available to all women and their babies.

CNMs may provide care in diverse settings, including homes, hospitals, birth centers, and a variety of ambulatory care settings, including private offices and community and public health clinics (APRN, 2008). CNMs' productivity is typically reported by outpatient visits, relative value units, and a combination of deliveries. The CNMs, physicians, and leadership may have set productivity targets based on internal or external benchmarks.

CNMs are less likely to be employed by the hospital, but they still impact your staffing. Consider the research findings that demonstrate:

- Low-risk women whose births were attended by CNMs had lower odds of a cesarean birth, induction/augmentation of labor, complications of birth, postpartum hemorrhage, endometritis, and preterm birth and higher odds of a vaginal birth, vaginal birth after cesarean, and breast-feeding than women whose births were attended by physicians (Hamlin et al., 2021).

- Regions with higher levels of nurse midwifery integration are associated with significantly higher rates of physiologic birth, less obstetric interventions, and fewer adverse neonatal outcomes (Vedam et al., 2018).

Here is the potential impact of CNMs on staffing:

- Lower cesarean section rates will require different RN staffing levels to care for patients who deliver naturally.

- Lower cesarean section rates will decrease and change your need for staffing your OB operating and recovery rooms differently.

- CNMs tend to do more underwater deliveries. Facilitate structural changes to support their practice and ensure staff competency.

- Lower cesarean section rates will decrease your delivery time and length of stay, requiring you to determine new RN staffing levels and patterns.

CNMs can have a positive impact on your patients' outcomes. This may require a change in your RN staffing and scheduling to meet the needs of more natural deliveries and fewer cesarean sections.

Certified Registered Nurse Anesthetists

The certified registered nurse anesthetist (CRNA) is prepared to provide the full spectrum of patients' anesthesia care and anesthesia-related care for individuals across their life span (APRN, 2008). This care can be provided in diverse settings, including hospital surgical suites and obstetrical delivery rooms, Critical Access Hospitals, acute care facilities, pain-management centers, ambulatory surgical centers, and other outpatient settings (APRN, 2008).

As with all APRNs, there has been concern from the medical establishment regarding the safety of the care provided. Research on CRNAs has found no statistically significant difference in mortality rates for CRNAs and anesthesiologists (Pine et al., 2003). Additionally, CRNAs are more accessible to vulnerable populations and rural areas (Vitale, 2021).

Most importantly, in a Cochrane review, researchers studying anesthesia safety found no differences in care between nurse anesthetists and physicians based on an exhaustive analysis of research literature published in the United States and worldwide (Lewis et al., 2014).

Here is the potential impact of CRNAs on staffing:

- Improved pain control through pain committee involvement leads to standardized pain protocols that give the RN a ready-to-use resource and may reduce the RN workload of managing pain by decreasing phone calls to other providers for orders.

- Improved pain control through proactive assessment and management between the CRNA and RN reduces RN workload, as the amount of time spent getting the patient's pain level to an acceptable level is decreased.

- Having the CRNAs and recovery-room staff start patients on patient-controlled analgesia (PCA) before coming to the floor decreases the workload of floor RNs.

CRNAs can have a positive impact on your patients and your staff. By working collaboratively with your CRNAs, you can decrease your RNs' workload for managing pain by having a proactive process to address it.

Quality-Management Staff

The background and licensure of quality-management staff vary. Some may be RNs, and some may hold additional certifications. Quality-management staff members significantly impact your unit based on their knowledge of quality, particularly core measures. *Core measures* are a set of inpatient and outpatient quality measures that help the organization improve its care. These measures are collected by most hospitals in the US and are reported on the CMS Hospital Compare website. Ask your quality manager for the measures that impact your unit.

TIP

For those who do not currently have core measures, measures are updated, revised, added, and removed regularly. Watch organizations like the National Quality Forum (NQF) to understand the direction quality might take. CMS adopts many of its recommendations. NQF announced in 2023 that it will join the Joint Commission enterprise, while maintaining its independence in convening and developing consensus-based measures, implementation guidance, and practices that benefit all stakeholders. NQF will continue to focus on accelerating widespread use of high-impact, low-burden measures that achieve affordable improvements in health for all.

With a value-based purchasing program in full swing, everyone is responsible for ensuring your organization's ability to meet CMS core measure goals. *Value-based purchasing* is a program in which CMS rewards or penalizes hospitals for quality measures. If you do not meet your organization's targets (set by CMS) for your care measures, your organization can lose money—millions each year. You might say, "My unit does not directly impact or own a core measure, so why should I care?" Not meeting value-based purchasing core-measure goals affects your whole organization, not just the units that directly impact the measures. The more your organization is penalized, the less money your organization has, and the effect will trickle down to your unit and negatively affect your budget.

> **NOTE**
>
> *Core measures are national standards of care for common conditions. Not all core measures are part of the current value-based purchasing methodology. The current method includes a sample of core and patient-satisfaction measures (Hospital Consumer Assessment of Healthcare Providers and Systems, or HCAHPS), weighted more toward the core measures.*

What does this have to do with staffing? For many core measures, nurses are doing the tasks, such as removing the Foley catheter in time or giving the last IV antibiotic—and documenting it. Furthermore, if something is not documented, it is not done, particularly regarding core measures. Some hospitals require unit staff to keep track of their own measures, while others have quality staff collect this data.

Here are things to consider with quality-management or quality improvement staff related to your staffing:

- Without QM staff, the RN may spend more time documenting and away from patient care.

- Rushed documentation can lead to misses in your organization's data.

- Staff needed to educate and evaluate knowledge of core-measure definition changes.

- Staff members must know the importance of completing specific tasks on time or within a certain time frame, including documentation, such as removing the Foley within 24 hours (not 24½ hours).

- Many patients impacting core measures on your unit may necessitate a more hybrid care delivery model that may include parts of a functional nursing care delivery model to ensure you meet your measure targets.

- QM staff can evaluate and make recommendations on areas for improvement in care on your unit while reducing healthcare costs.

Having dedicated quality staff to assist with education and data collection means less for your staff to do and may help improve productivity. Depending on your core-measure outcomes, it may support hiring more quality specialists to improve those quality scores.

Case Managers

Case management is a constantly evolving role. The American Case Management Association (ACMA) defines case management as:

> a dynamic process that assesses, plans, implements, coordinates, monitors, and evaluates to improve outcomes, experiences, and value. The practice of case management is professional and collaborative, occurring in a variety of settings where medical care, mental health care, and social support are delivered. Services are facilitated by diverse disciplines in conjunction with the care recipient and their support system. In pursuit of health equity, priorities include identifying needs, ensuring appropriate access to resources/services, addressing social determinants of health, and facilitating safe care transitions. Professional case managers help navigate complex systems to achieve mutual goals, advocate for those they serve, and recognize personal dignity, autonomy, and the right to self-determination. (ACMA, 2020, p. 2)

Most direct care RNs and many managers need to understand the complete role of a case manager on their unit and the impact of case managers on length of stay and staffing. The staff often underutilizes the RN and MSW case manager in dealing with a complex patient with high needs. Alternatively, the direct care RNs' and managers' efforts at discharge planning for their patients overlap with the case manager's role in discharge planning. Because case managers typically report centrally, unit management may need to be more aware of these individuals' full role, skills, and abilities. You must know the case managers on your unit (and their boss) and ensure you effectively work together to maximize their skills and your staff's time.

Case managers typically are RNs or licensed medical social workers (MSWs). Hospital case management can differ greatly from community case management, transitional care management, and even insurance case management. Hospital case managers aim to ensure high-quality patient care and hospital outcomes, efficient resource utilization, and reimbursement for services. Typical case-management staffing ratios are 1:18–20 case managers to patients, but they depend on the model and job functions and additional resources they have, including social workers.

High-functioning case management departments (often referred to care management departments in hospitals) function with a triad model (or collaborative model) of RNs, MSWs, and assistive staff. Functions are divided such that both the RN and the MSW practice to the highest level of their license. This looks like the RNs overseeing the medical portions of a discharge plan partnering with the MSW who is overseeing the psychosocial aspects of the discharge. They are partnered with an assistant who can fax paperwork to insurances and post-acute agencies, as well as make appointments.

Consider This

The hours that the case management office is open, and staff are available are very important in improving outcomes. Hospitals discharge patients 24/7, so is your case management staff available every day, including the weekend? Research shows that 30-day readmission rates are higher for those patients discharged on the weekend (Chiu et al., 2020). What is your staffing (including case management) coverage over the weekends? Lack of additional staff, services, and management can have a negative impact on patient outcomes.

Within a hospital setting, case managers perform many functions including but not limited to (ACMA, 2020):

- Collaborate with patients/families/caregivers in goal setting that is reflective of the location of care.

- Utilize a validated system/defined methodology for tracking avoidable delays/days as well as over/under utilization of resources. This information will be used to identify and communicate opportunities for improvement.

- Proactively prevent medical necessity denials by providing education to physicians, staff, and patients, interfacing with payers and documenting relevant information.

- Promote and facilitate care delivery for the setting and duration that is appropriate to the clinical need.

- Provide information to the healthcare team, patient/family/caregiver regarding available resources and benefits for services across the continuum that ensures patient choice, safety, and timeliness with each transition.

- Advocate for the patient while balancing the responsibility of stewardship for their organization, and in general, the judicious management of resources.

Here are things to consider related to the impact of case managers on staffing:

- Do you and your staff know the high-risk screening tools used by case managers to identify your high-risk patients? How are they defined?

- Ensure that your definition and understanding of a high-risk patient are identical to theirs.

- Implement interdisciplinary rounds that include your staff RN and case managers (and others) to discuss daily patient progression.

- Educate your staff on how and when to contact the case manager to assist in discharge or transition needs.

- Develop and ensure resources for your staff RNs who must facilitate the discharge of complex patients for off times instead of keeping a patient over a weekend.

- Based on your unit's volume, consider case management services/coverage on evenings or weekends to facilitate patient flow and decrease workload and staffing needs for your unit's RNs.

- Create a process where case managers facilitate discharges prior to the weekend. Decreased patient volume on the weekend may decrease your staff's need to work weekends, such as every third weekend versus every other.

Case managers are essential in facilitating patient flow and discharges for your unit. Complex patient discharges can take a significant amount of your staff's time and can increase workload and staffing needs, especially in the absence of case-management resources.

Pharmacists

Pharmacies within hospitals differ considerably from community pharmacies. This difference dramatically influences your pharmacist's role in the hospital and your unit, which varies from hospital to hospital. Due to the nature of acute care versus community, the pharmacist in the hospital setting may have more complex clinical medication–management issues while providing medication and nutritional consults (Hammond et al., 2019).

Clinical pharmacy is defined by the American College of Clinical Pharmacy (ACCP) as, "a health science discipline in which pharmacists provide patient care that optimizes medication therapy and promotes health, wellness, and disease prevention" (ACCP, 2020, para. 2). Clinical pharmacists, those practicing in the hospital setting, specialize in a specific area, such as hematology/oncology, HIV/AIDS, infectious disease, critical care, emergency medicine, toxicology, nuclear pharmacy, pain management, psychiatry, anticoagulation clinics, herbal medicine, neurology/epilepsy management, pediatrics, or neonatology (Burke et al., 2008). Pharmacist productivity for a decentralized model will depend on their workload, which includes such components as verification of orders, discontinuation of orders, patient-profile review, preparation of progress notes, contribution to the patient-care plan, consultation, attendance at interdisciplinary unit rounds, reporting of unexpected medication events, and responses to emergency resuscitation codes.

Here are things to consider related to pharmacist staffing:

- A decentralized pharmacist model and a pharmacist assigned to your unit will decrease RN workload and medication errors as the pharmacist assists or owns the medication-reconciliation process.

- Include the pharmacist with patients, nurses, and physicians in your interdisciplinary rounding process to improve communication related to patients' medication regimens and resolve medication issues in real time.

- The pharmacist can work with staff to optimize the patient's medication, including monitoring and decreasing inappropriate or overuse of proton pump inhibitor medications that have been shown to increase hospital-acquired infections (HAIs) such as C. difficile. Increased HAI increases the length of patient stay and your RNs' workload through the additional need to gown up each time they enter that patient's room.

- The pharmacist can facilitate the transition of patients from IV to PO medications and antibiotics faster, decreasing the time RNs spend administering and monitoring time-consuming IV antibiotics.

- Even without a decentralized pharmacist model, include the pharmacist as the lead or a member in the medication-reconciliation process.

- A pharmacist on the unit can assist providers in ordering the right drug and decrease the time staff spend administering a less-than-optimal medication or time spent by staff on the phone reconciling this issue (ACCP, 2020).

- Have the pharmacist create a comprehensive drug therapy plan for patients. This can improve RNs' ability to ensure and facilitate discharge with the proper medications (Burke et al., 2008).

Clinical pharmacists are trained to resolve medication nonadherence issues through comprehensive medication management (CMM; Brummel et al., 2016). In a team-based care approach, pharmacists assist in managing medication therapy problems such as inadequate therapy, nonadherence, adverse reactions, unnecessary therapy, and dosing that is too high (Brummel et al., 2016). Pharmacists can positively impact RN staffing by decreasing RN workload around medication use, appropriateness, and administration, whether in a centralized or decentralized model.

Pharmacists can also enhance patient outcomes through, for example, improving medication adherence and reducing the possibility of HAI.

Healthcare Social Work

Healthcare social work (often still referred to as medical social work in some states) is a sub-discipline of social work. MSWs can be employed in many healthcare settings and play a vital role on an interprofessional team. They may be different than clinical social workers in your state. These individuals can provide psychosocial support to people, families, or vulnerable populations so they can cope with chronic, acute, or terminal illnesses, such as Alzheimer's disease, cancer, or AIDS. They also advise family caregivers, counsel patients, and help plan for patients' needs after discharge from hospitals (National Association of Social Workers [NASW], 2023). A master's degree in social work is typically required for positions in health settings and clinical work (NASW, 2023).

MSWs play a vital role in patient flow in your unit. Delays in patient discharge will increase your unit's length of stay, increase resource usage, and decrease net revenue. MSWs work collaboratively with case managers in many hospitals to facilitate patient discharge.

The MSW's role can include (NASW, 2023):

- Working with patients and their families in need of psychosocial help
- Assessing the psychosocial functioning of patients and families and intervening as necessary
- Connecting patients and families to necessary resources and support in the community
- Providing psychotherapy, supportive counseling, or grief counseling
- Helping a patient expand and strengthen their network of social supports

- Collaborating in the development of a discharge plan that will meet the patient's needs and allow the patient to leave the hospital in a timely manner

MSWs also can quickly and effectively establish a therapeutic relationship with patients. Behavioral health patients can become a time burden and increase safety risks, especially if you are not a behavioral health unit. Due to a lack of appropriate behavioral health services in many communities, your staff may face more behavioral health patients needing acute care medical or surgical services. MSWs, mainly when behavioral health nurses and staff are absent, may improve your staff's safety, decrease restraint usage, reduce staffing costs, and improve productivity.

MSW Behavioral Health Intervention

We had a patient admitted to a suicide attempt, and as he was not medically clear, he was admitted to the floors. Once on the unit, plans were made to transfer him to a psychiatric facility. The patient became quite belligerent, and security was called. The patient was shouting that he was "special forces" and would take out the three security officers preparing to restrain him. We were able to have the officers withdraw and, with assistance from social work, de-escalate the patient to the point that we could provide a safe transfer.

–Thomas Aronson, MBA, LCSW

Here are things to consider related to MSWs and staffing:

- Clarify the process for your staff on when to call for a social work evaluation. Your RN staff do not need to do everything themselves; they need to utilize all the available resources.

- Understand the social work department's process and criteria for assessing high-risk patients. Opportunities may exist to teach your staff or work with MSWs to improve their support service to your unit based on individual unit needs.

- Provide patient behavioral health support, which may decrease your RNs' workload. This may be more important if your organization or community lacks sufficient behavioral health resources and placement agencies.

- Include the MSW in interdisciplinary rounds. Clarify for your staff and other disciplines the role of the MSW and the role of the case manager, which may overlap slightly and confuse some staff members, decreasing their comfort in requesting help from these resources.

- Post weekend and after-hours coverage of MSWs for your staff to help manage patients as needed. Weekend and night RNs may feel they have few or no resources for help and may attempt to take over the role of another individual to give the patient the care they believe is needed. This increases the workload of the RN.

MSWs can provide your staff with a wide range of support services, from assistance in patient discharges and social or financial barriers to behavioral health support.

Chaplains

There are many types of chaplains, including healthcare, military, and prison, just to name a few. Chaplains assist with patients', families', and staff's pastoral, spiritual, and emotional needs. Healthcare chaplains are usually highly educated, board-certified members of the interdisciplinary team. Education usually includes a Master of Divinity; board certification requires additional training in clinical pastoral education. Although some hospitals have worked with their community's pastors and chaplains to rotate through a volunteer schedule to cover a hospital's needs, other hospitals may employ chaplains or even serve as a place for chaplain residencies. The number of chaplains needed per hospital may vary as there is no consensus on what services should be provided by a spiritual services department (Tartaglia, Corson, et al., 2024). Research supports the notion that staffing levels are a function of chaplain integration into an organization and the activities organizations expect chaplains to fulfill (Tartaglia, Corson, et al., 2024). One study of 93 pediatric hospitals found an average of 2.1 chaplains per average of 171 beds (Wintz & Handzo, 2005).

Many managers, hospitals, and staff need to pay more attention to the value chaplains place on the patient's experience. Also, many nurses feel unable to meet patients' spiritual needs due to their discomfort with discussing spirituality or religion. In addition to discomfort, the RN may not feel prepared to discuss or support a patient's spiritual needs. One study found that chaplains increase the enrollment of patients into hospice care (Flannelly et al., 2012). This will free up beds in your unit and decrease your staff's workload by moving patients to the right level of service. Post COVID-19, with nurses' increased levels of moral distress, consider using chaplain services for staff issues, such as a death or severe accident. In one study, chaplains at over half of the hospitals spent an estimated 10% to 30% of their time on staff care, with chaplains in five hospitals spending greater than 30% (Tartaglia, White, et al., 2024)

Here are things to consider related to the impact of chaplains on staffing:

- Determine the highest need times for your patients with chaplain services. Ensure your staff RNs know when the chaplains are available or are on call and how to contact them.

- In addition to the initial assessment questions concerning their spiritual and religious needs, work with your staff and chaplains to ensure appropriate follow-up with the patient to see whether needs have changed.

- Ensure that your staff knows the chaplain's role and when they can be contacted, such as in family and patient conflict regarding DNR status.

- Involve the chaplain in the interdisciplinary rounding process to allow them to assess for potential chaplain services or needs.

- Post the times for worship services.

- Educate your staff on how chaplains support patients of all faiths and beliefs and how they can assist in finding further support in that patient's religion through their contact list.

- Encourage chaplains to educate staff on different faiths and beliefs to improve their comfort level with discussions of religion and spirituality.

Chaplains' integration into the healthcare team improves patients' satisfaction with their hospital stay (Marin et al., 2015). As well, a study by Wall and associates (2007) noted that family members of a patient who died in the ICU or 24 hours after discharge were more likely to say they were satisfied with the spiritual care they received if a pastor or spiritual advisor was involved in the last 24 hours of the patient's life. Additionally, a strong association exists between satisfaction with spiritual care and satisfaction with the total ICU experience (Wall et al., 2007). Chaplains offer a beneficial service to patients and staff that can improve the patient experience and decrease the workload of their staff by using all available resources.

Respiratory Therapists

Respiratory therapists (RTs) are healthcare practitioners who treat patients with respiratory and cardiac issues and specialize in the promotion of optimal cardiopulmonary function and health (Kacmarek et al., 2019). Many RTs work closely with pulmonologists and can perform and are specialists in (Harbrecht et al., 2009):

- Airway management—actively maintaining an open airway during the management of trauma

- Administering anesthesia for surgery or conscious sedation

- Initiating and managing life support for people in intensive care units and emergency departments

- Stabilizing and monitoring high-risk patients being moved from hospital to hospital by air or ground ambulance

- Administering inhaled drugs and medical gases, such as asthma medication, oxygen, and anesthetic gases

- Conducting tests to measure lung function and teaching people to manage their respiratory condition

RTs as Part of the Vascular Access Team

Due to a nursing shortage and a decreased availability of physicians, central line placement needed to be faster to facilitate timely care. Because there was no shortage of RTs, a pilot was developed to educate them to place central lines under the order and supervision of a physician. An important step was obtaining a position from Arizona's Board of Respiratory Care Examiners. The board stated:

> As previously established, central line insertion is considered part of the Respiratory Care scope of practice based on the interpretation of the law, given the practitioner has received appropriate advanced training, participates in timely continuing education/ skill reevaluation, and is performing under medical direction. After a Respiratory Care Practitioner has met the training and competency standards as previously stated, preceptorship is at the discretion of hospital policy. (Arizona State Board of Respiratory Care, 2009, p. 4)

After meeting the requests of the board and developing hospital policy, procedures, and standards, a pilot was conducted to determine the results. Results showed outcomes of insertion and infection rates to be the same as the physician-placed lines.

–Jennifer Mensik-Kennedy, PhD, MBA, RN, NEA-BC, FAAN

Here are things to consider related to the impact of RTs on staffing:

- RTs are valuable to the rapid response and/or code team.
- Ensure the RT attends your unit's interdisciplinary rounds.
- Complete education and clarify when and what respiratory care the RT provides and when the RN may provide it.
- Cross-train and expand the role of the RT to help meet the needs of your unit, which may include completing EKGs and inserting or maintaining central and PICC lines.

- Clarify the role of the RT on your unit for night and day shifts and weekends. If your staff RNs perceive no support, they will attempt to do everything instead of contacting the appropriate resource for help. Getting RT support may decrease RNs' workload.

RTs' productivity is typically measured by RVUs (Relative Value Units) or some combination of RVUs and other measurements. Strict RVUs may not equal a good measure of productivity because not all RT activities have a corresponding CPT code that will translate into an RVU. A few examples of activities without CPT codes that are critical to producing good outcomes and for which your organization may require an RT include (1) spontaneous breathing trials for ventilator patients, (2) rapid response calls when patients are in respiratory distress, and (3) participation in high-risk deliveries. These components are essential in considering the staffing needs of RTs in conjunction with your RN needs.

NOTE

RTs provide traditional respiratory services but have expanded their role and scope in many areas. Utilize all staff to their ability to decrease the workload and needs of your RN staff.

Hospitalists

Hospitalists include physicians, physician associates (what were known as physician assistants [PAs]), and nurse practitioners whose primary focus is hospital medicine. A 2020 report shares that over 83% of hospital medicine groups employ NPs and PAs (Kaplan & Klein, 2021). A hospitalist is different from an intensivist, whose focus is intensive care. However, hospitalists partner with intensivists and all other specialists, including the primary care provider, to treat patients. In this vein, hospitalists act as care coordinators among the other specialty physicians and surgeons for a patient. Hospitalists may also be leaders on various teams and quality champions for ensuring hospital-required quality measures in their control are met.

This medical specialty has developed significantly in recent years, as many primary care physicians (PCPs) prefer to stay in their clinics where they can generate more revenue. Many PCPs would see patients in the evening, contributing to longer lengths of stay as hospital staff waited all day for the physician to come in, see the patient, and write orders to advance care. Hospital leadership saw the need to decrease lengths of stay and improve quality. Hospital reimbursement continues to be cut, and mandated hospital quality measures are constantly changing, but these were not a high priority for the PCP. Hospitalists typically do not have a practice outside the hospital; however, they may provide medical oversight post-discharge to patients who do not have a primary care provider or have yet to see that provider for a short duration of time after discharge. Research does show that hospitalists' patients have a decreased length of stay and increased patient satisfaction when compared with non-hospitalists (Salim et al., 2019).

A hospitalist's productivity is typically measured in RVUs.

Here are things to consider related to the impact of hospitalists on staffing:

- Hospitalist availability means your staff has faster access to a provider who can write orders.

- The medical plan of patient care progresses faster, so you may need to work with your RNs to match the nursing plan-of-care progress to the medical progression. Also, educate your RNs that although a patient may be medically discharged, they do need to finish and meet the nursing needs and goals of the patient, which are just as important.

- Understand the hospitalists' schedules, assigned units, and rounding process. Ask your staff to consolidate questions for the hospitalist and, if possible, to wait until the hospitalist arrives at the unit. Additional phone calls from other units will decrease the hospitalist's ability to see patients in a timely manner.

- Based on the needs of your unit (and organization) and patient population, there may be a need for a night hospitalist to facilitate care, which will decrease the workload for your RNs and improve their ability to provide timely care.

- Structure interdisciplinary rounds so that the hospitalist can attend.

- Understand which quality measures the hospitalist is responsible for.

Hospitalists are relatively new to the healthcare team and are growing in numbers as a specialty. As an onsite provider for medical orders, a hospitalist can help your staff give timely care while improving patient care and decreasing RN workload.

Residents

Residents provide a valued service to many hospitals in providing around-the-clock care to their patient population, typically in a teaching or academic hospital. A resident is a graduate of medical school. Residencies give the graduate in-depth training within a specific branch of medicine. Residents, like hospitalists, are always available to see patients and can improve the flow of your unit. However, residents are still training, so they may rely on your more senior nursing staff when handling complex medical patients.

Here are things to consider related to the impact of residents on staffing:

- With their role on the care team, invite them to your unit's interdisciplinary rounds.

- Clarify the process for staff in determining the call schedule when multiple residents are on the floor.

- Understand their education schedule and process for rounding with their faculty. If there is no straightforward process or time for this, work with the faculty to provide some schedule. This will improve your staff's access to an ordering provider and decrease the number of phones calls and pages the RNs make to them.

- Clarify the chain of command for your staff members if they do not agree with something the resident orders. Staff members must feel comfortable escalating their concerns to managers, the department chair, or the attending physician. (Hospitals may or may not consider the resident the attending.)

- Because residents' schedules rotate, tell your staff when new residents come onto the unit. Nothing will slow down your staff more than paging a resident who is no longer on rotation in your department and unit. With residents and many teaching hospitals, the length of stay for comparable community-type patients may be longer. Make sure you consider this when staffing and scheduling.

Residents are valuable members of the healthcare team in academic and teaching hospitals. Due to the nature of their education and rotating schedules, ensure that your staff is educated to work collaboratively within this model of care.

Summary

Here are the key points covered in this chapter:

- Many other professionals impact your unit and staffing.
- Understand the scope and role of all individuals caring for patients.
- Delineate the roles of other professionals and ensure that your nursing staff understands these roles.
- Utilize other disciplines to their full potential, ability, and scope to provide patient care.
- Staff RNs do not need to provide all aspects of patient care.
- Utilizing all disciplines and creating a true interdisciplinary partnership will decrease your staff RNs' workload and improve your patients' quality and satisfaction.

References

Aiken, L. H., Sloane, D. M., Brom, H. M., Todd, B. A., Barnes, H., Cimiotti, J. P., Cunningham, R. S., & McHugh, M. D. (2021). Value of nurse practitioner inpatient hospital staffing. *Medical Care, 59*(10), 857–863. https://doi.org/10.1097/MLR.0000000000001628

American Case Management Association. (2020). *Case management standards of practice & scope of services.* https://www.acmaweb.org/forms/Standards_of%20Practice_Scope_of%20 Services_Brochure.pdf

American College of Clinical Pharmacy. (2020). *Definition of clinical pharmacy.* https://www. accp.com/stunet/compass/definition.aspx

American College of Nurse-Midwives. (2019). *ACNM Core Data Survey 2019.* www.midwife. org/acnm/files/cclibraryfiles/filename/000000008291/ACNM%202019%20Core%20Data%20 Survey%20Report.pdf

APRN Consensus Work Group & the National Council of State Boards of Nursing APRN Advisory Committee. (2008, July 7). *Consensus model for APRN regulation: Licensure, accreditation, certification & education.* APRN Joint Dialogue Group Report. https://www. nursingworld.org/~4aa7d9/globalassets/certification/aprn_consensus_model_report_7-7-08.pdf

Arizona State Board of Respiratory Care. (2009, March 19). *Examiners board meeting minutes.* https://respiratoryboard.az.gov/sites/default/files/2022-03/2009-3-19_0.pdf

Brummel, A., & Carlson, A. M. (2016). Comprehensive medication management and medication adherence for chronic conditions. *Journal of Managed Care & Specialty Pharmacy, 22*(1), 56–62. https://doi.org/10.18553/jmcp.2016.22.1.56

Burke, J. M., Miller, W. A., Spencer, A. P., Crank, C. W., Adkins, L., Bertch, K. E., Ragucci, D. P., Smith, W. E., & Valley, A. W. (2008). Clinical pharmacist competencies. *Pharmacotherapy, 28*(6), 806–815. https://doi.org/10.1592/phco.28.6.806

Chiu, C.-Y., Oria, D., Yangga, P., & Kang, D. (2020). Quality assessment of weekend discharge: A systematic review and meta-analysis. *International Journal for Quality in Health Care, 32*(6), 347–355. https://doi.org/10.1093/intqhc/mzaa060

Federal Trade Commission. (2014, March). *Policy perspectives: Competition and the regulation of advanced practice nurses.* https://www.ftc.gov/reports/policy-perspectives-competition-regulation-advanced-practice-nurses

Fikre, R., Gubbels, J., Teklesilasie, W., & Gerards, S. (2023). Effectiveness of midwifery-led care on pregnancy outcomes in low- and middle-income countries: A systematic review and meta-analysis. *BMC Pregnancy Childbirth, 23*(1), 386. https://doi: 10.1186/ s12884-023-05664-9

Flannelly, K. J., Emanuel, L. L., Handzo, G. F., Galek, K., Silton, N. R., & Carlson, M. (2012). A national study of chaplaincy services and end of life outcomes. *BMC Palliative Care, 11*(10), 1–6. https://doi.org/10.1186/1472-684X-11-10

Gershengorn, H. B., Wunsch, H., Wahab, R., Leaf, D. E., Brodie, D., Li, G., & Factor, P. (2011). Impact of nonphysician staffing on outcomes in a medical ICU. *Chest, 139*(6), 1347–1353. https://doi.org/10.1378/chest.10-2648

Hamlin, L., Grunwald, L., Sturdivant, R. X., & Koehlmoos, T. P. (2021). Comparison of nurse-midwife and physician birth outcomes in the military health system. *Policy, Politics, & Nursing Practice, 22*(2), 105–113. https://doi.org/10.1177/1527154421994071

Hammond, D. A., Flowers, H. J., Meena, N., Painter, J. T., & Rech, M. A. (2019). Cost avoidance associated with clinical pharmacist presence in a medical intensive care unit. *Journal of the American College of Clinical Pharmacy, 2*(6), 610–615. https://doi.org/10.1002/jac5.1111

Harbrecht, B. G., Delgado, E., Tuttle, R. P., Cohen-Melamed, M. H., Saul, M. I., & Valenta, C. A. (2009). Improved outcomes with routine respiratory therapist evaluation of non-intensive-care-unit surgery patients. *Respiratory Care, 54*(7), 861–867. https://doi.org/10.4187/002013209793800457

Hays, V. (2010). Pressure ulcer prevention and treatment program: Successful strategies implanted by a med/surg clinical nurse specialist. *Clinical Nurse Specialist, 24*(2), 99–100. https://doi.org/10.1097/01.NUR.0000348948.36446.a6

Kacmarek, R. M., Stoller, J. K., & Heuer, A. J. (2019). *Egan's fundamentals of respiratory care e-book.* Elsevier Health Sciences.

Kaplan, L., & Klein, T. (2021). Nurse practitioner hospitalists: An empowered role. *Nursing Outlook, 69*(5), 856–864. https://doi.org/10.1016/j.outlook.2021.03.015

The Lancet. (2014, June 23). Midwifery matters 'more than ever,' experts say. *ScienceDaily.* www.sciencedaily.com/releases/2014/06/140623092938.htm

Lewis, S. R., Nicholson, A., Smith, A. F., & Alderson, P. (2014, July). Physician anaesthetists versus non-physician providers of anaesthesia for surgical patients. *Cochrane Database of Systematic Reviews.* http://onlinelibrary.wiley.com/doi/10.1002/14651858.CD010357.pub2/full

Liu, C. F., Hebert, P. L., Douglas, J. H., Neely, E. L., Sulc, C. A., Reddy, A., Sales, A. E., & Wong, E. S. (2020). Outcomes of primary care delivery by nurse practitioners: Utilization, cost, and quality of care. *Health Services Research, 55*(2), 178–189. https://doi.org/10.1111/1475-6773.13246

Marin, D. B., Sharma, V., Sosunov, E., Egorova, N., Goldstein, R., & Handzo, G. F. (2015). Relationship between chaplain visits and patient satisfaction. *Journal of Health Care Chaplaincy, 21*(1), 14–24. https://doi.org/10.1080/08854726.2014.981417

National Association of Social Workers. (2023). *Who are social workers?* https://www.socialworkers.org/News/Facts/Social-Workers

Newhouse, R., Stanik-Hutt, J., White, K. M., Johantgen, M., Bass, E. B., Zangaro, G., Wilson, R. F., Steinwachs, D. M., Heindel, L., & Weiner, J. P. (2011). Advanced practice nurse outcomes 1990–2008: A systematic review. *Nursing Economic$, 29*(5), 230–250.

Office of Technology Assessment. (1981). *The cost and effectiveness of nurse practitioners.* US Government Printing Office.

Pajerski, D., Harlan, M., Ren, D., & Tuite, P. K. (2022). A clinical nurse specialist–led initiative to reduce catheter-associated urinary tract infection rates using a best practice guideline. *Clinical Nurse Specialist, 36*(1), 20–28. https://doi.org/10.1097/NUR.0000000000000643

Pine, M., Holt, K. D., & Lou, Y. B. (2003). Surgical mortality and type of anesthesia provider. *American Association of Nurse Anesthetists Journal, 71,* 109–116.

Richardson, J., & Tjoelker, R. (2012). Beyond the central line-associated bloodstream infection bundle: The value of the clinical nurse specialist in continuing evidence-based practice changes. *Clinical Nurse Specialist, 26*(4), 205–211. https://doi.org/10.1097/NUR.0b013e31825aebab

Salim, S. A., Elmaraezy, A., Pamarthy, A., Thongprayoon, C., Cheungpasitporn, W., & Palabindala, V. (2019). Impact of hospitalists on the efficiency of inpatient care and patient satisfaction: A systematic review and meta-analysis. *Journal of Community Hospital Internal Medicine Perspectives, 9*(2), 121–134. https://doi.org/10.1080/20009666.2019.1591901

Tartaglia, A., Corson, T., White, K. B., Charlescraft, A., Jackson-Jordan, E., Johnson, T., & Fitchett, G. (2024). Chaplain staffing and scope of service: Benchmarking spiritual care departments. *Journal of Health Care Chaplaincy, 30*(1), 1–18. https://doi.org/10.1080/08854726.2022.2121579

Tartaglia, A., White, K. B., Corson, T., Charlescraft, A., Johnson, T., Jackson-Jordan, E., & Fitchett, G. (2024). Supporting staff: The role of health care chaplains. *Journal of Health Care Chaplaincy, 30*(1), 60–73. https://doi.org/10.1080/08854726.2022.2154107

Vedam, S., Stoll, K., MacDorman, M., Declercq, E., Cramer, R., Cheyney, M., Fisher, T., Butt, E., Yang, Y. T., & Kennedy, H. P. (2018). Mapping integration of midwives across the United States: Impact on access, equity, and outcomes. *PLoS ONE, 13*(2), e0192523. https://doi.org/10.1371/journal.pone.0192523

Vitale, C. M., & Lyons, K. S. (2021). The state of nurse anesthetist practice and policy: An integrative review. *AANA Journal, 89*(5), 403–412.

Wall, R. J., Engelberg, R. A., Gries, C. J., Glavan, B., & Curtis, J. R. (2007). Spiritual care of families in the intensive care unit. *Critical Care Medicine, 35*(4), 1084–1090. https://doi.org/10.1097/01.CCM.0000259382.36414.06

Wintz, S., & Handzo, G. (2005). Pastoral care staffing and productivity: More than ratios. *Chaplaincy Today, 21*(1), 3–10. https://doi.org/10.1080/10999183.2005.10767268

Recognize, Manage, and Minimize Your Variability

This may come as a shock to you, but most nurses think their patients are different—different from patients in a similar unit in a neighboring hospital or in another state. Your patients *are* different in the sense that no two people are the same. What you want to chalk up to patient differences is due to artificial and natural variability. These "variable traits" make it difficult, if not impossible, to manage if you do not know what they are.

So, let us start with the premise that your patients are unique and different. But let us also start with the fact that you can manage and eliminate variability that impacts your unit. In this chapter, we discuss the two types of variability, what variability means for you, what control you may or may not have over it, and how you can staff your unit with real information and data.

One Size Does Not Fit All

Healthcare organizations, particularly hospitals, are complex systems. And no two systems are exactly alike, even within the same healthcare system. What works for one will not work for everyone. For example, what works in one emergency department (ED) may not work in another. But, although some things are not in our control, others are. Focus on what you can change, not what you cannot. As we discuss variability, what variables might impact your unit and make it different?

- Culture?

- Community?

- Socioeconomics?

- Case mix index of patients?

- Historical patient volumes?

- Clinical staff vacancy?

These are the things that really make each of our units different.

The Ebb and Flow of Your Department

Some refer to the natural movement of a unit in their hospital as the ebb and flow, or valleys and peaks, or patient flow. Whatever you call it, that movement typically reflects the coming and going of patients, and it has a major impact on your staffing. From a more scientific perspective, this "movement" is called *variability*.

Before the change in reimbursement of the 1980s and 1990s, hospital administrators staffed nurses based on the number of beds, not necessarily whether those beds were being used. Nursing represents the single largest cost to a hospital, so as reimbursement changed, hospital administrators attempted to control costs by matching nursing resources to average census. The problem with this method occurs when patient volumes peak in excess of the average. For example, a peak in your census may be considered a 15% to 40% increase above your mean, or average, census.

> ## Consider This
>
> Each additional patient per nurse was associated with a 7% increase in the likelihood of dying within 30 days of admission and a 7% increase in the odds of failure to rescue (Aiken et al., 2002).

Daily fluctuations in census can be as much as 30% to 50% or more depending on the unit type. Staffing to the peak is too costly, staffing to the valleys is not safe, and staffing to the average does not take into consideration the peaks or valleys. The next logical thing is to control for as much of the variation as possible by smoothing the peaks and valleys (trying to create rolling hills instead). To do this, you need to actively manage and eliminate as much variability as you can. But first, you need to know what the potential sources of variability are.

There are two types of variability—artificial and natural—and each impacts your unit, some more than others. (Because one size does not fit all, there may be some things that impact your variability that are not discussed here.) First we review all types and subtypes of variability and discuss how you can manage or smooth them on your unit. The key for you to really impact your unit is to understand all your areas of variability. Let us begin by discussing artificial variability.

> ## Consider This
>
> When staffing to the average census, keep this in mind: Census increases up to 25% above an adequate (average) staffing level subject all patients in the nursing unit in question to a 7% increase in [mortality] risk (Litvak et al., 2005).

Artificial Variability

Artificial variability refers to the way we schedule services and allocate resources—thus, our inability to manage effectively our beds and staff. Dysfunctionally scheduled admissions is the most attributable cause of artificial variability, which can be decreased or eliminated by load smoothing (Asgari & Asgari, 2021). Elective surgeries and admissions often drive artificial variability. Smoothing surgical patient flow can improve hospital efficiency, the quality of care, and timely access to care for emergent and urgent surgeries (Litvak et al., 2021).

Surgery Schedule and the Impact on the Floor

You have experienced those days, usually at the beginning of the week, where it seems like there is a surgical patient needing a bed every minute. Then, the surgery schedule tapers out by the end of the week, and by Sunday afternoon, your unit is pretty quiet, a definite valley in your "average" census. All the while, Monday and Tuesday are lurking, with a surgical schedule waiting to wreak havoc on your unit again. This is the artificial variability that needs smoothing. Although you cannot really impact unscheduled surgeries, you (your organization) can do a better job of smoothing elective cases. If you are not a surgical manager, you may not know how "typical" surgery scheduling happens. Your hospital may schedule surgeries differently, or maybe it has managed or smoothed out this process already.

At most hospitals, surgeons or specialty groups (e.g., orthopedic or ear, nose, and throat specialists) are scheduled in blocks, which are fixed times on fixed days. You might find that certain surgeons "own" their blocks because they have the highest volume of patients who bring in the most money for the hospital. Or maybe the surgeon has a certain block due to their status in the community. Either way, smoothing surgeon schedules is not easy and will take an organizational approach that is data-driven, not emotion-driven. These blocks have an impact on your staffing. Underused blocks result in the valleys in surgical volume, for example, and blocks used beyond their fixed amount lead to the peaks in volume. You might need higher staffing on the weekends if you smooth the surgery schedule to have an increased volume on Friday, but you will have better patient outcomes, increased staff satisfaction, and gain operational efficiencies in all direct care and ancillary departments.

Consider This

Surgeons' blocked time (artificial variability) may be influenced by, or scheduled in tandem with, professional variability (discussed later). Surgeons may have other demands, such as teaching residents and their clinic hours. You have to work with the surgeons to redistribute surgery schedules or you might find the surgeon leaving for the next hospital with their patients.

So, what is the possible impact of artificial variability on patient flow and your RN staff? Say one day at your hospital, 30 scheduled surgery patients are admitted and tomorrow 50 are admitted, yet budgets staff for an average of 40 patients. The increased demand of 10 more surgical patients that one day increases demand and competition of scarce resources between scheduled admissions and other admissions, such as those through the ED and direct admits (Litvak, 2005). This competition leads to "nurse overload, understaffing, medical errors, and an undesirable work environment" (Litvak, 2005, p. 100) on those days with above-average demands, while it creates wasted capacity and wasted resources on those days with below-average demands.

Organize Work Differently

Other sources of artificial variability in your unit or organization may stem from how you organize work. How many times have you heard someone say, "That's the way we always do it here"? Does this mentality impact your variability? Does the way your unit or staff does things create unnecessary variability? For instance, if your case managers have a staff meeting daily at 2 p.m. during the same time as your interdisciplinary rounds, this artificial variability may hamper discharge-planning efforts and lead to decreased patient flow. In the last section of this chapter, on finding your own variability, you have a chance to think about this further.

> **Consider This**
>
> Another potential source of smoothing artificial variability is in the rounding practices of hospital physicians. The major cause of ED overcrowding is patients waiting for an inpatient bed and a lack of hospital capacity. Expanding ED capacity mainly increases ED boarding and continues to further overwhelm staff (McKenna et al., 2019). Build more hospital beds then, right? Not when the average cost is $1.5–$2 million per bed (Bazuin, 2010). The more logical first step is to look at physician practice and preference.
>
> Physicians typically start with the sickest patients to round on first, which means intensive care first, then progressive care/telemetry, followed by medical-surgical units. Why is this an issue? You typically cannot transfer patients to lower levels of care (or admit from the ED to ICU) until that medical-surgical patient goes home. And more than likely, the medical-surgical unit is full, too.
>
> Try having the physician round on the medical-surgical patients first, then have your unit discharge them soon thereafter. Physicians are always concerned about the more-acute ICU patient, but the more-acute patient also has a lot more nursing resources supporting their care.
>
> Another important strategy to smooth artificial variability that nurse leaders can impact is the discharge process. Including case management and/or social work early in the admission and creating a plan for discharge at the beginning of the hospital stay not only promotes engagement from the patient and family but also ensures that on the day of discharge the patient can leave as early as possible, promoting effective patient flow.

Natural Variability

Natural variability refers to the random factors that impact your unit. Although you cannot eliminate these random factors, you can manage them. There are three subtypes of natural variability: clinical, patient flow, and professional.

Clinical Variability

Clinical variability refers to the difference between each patient, such as symptoms, diseases, and socioeconomic factors. How do you manage clinical variability? Part of this answer is in managing patient flow in your ED, but another may be in how you organize your unit and hospital. You may have separate floors or units for cardiac patients and orthopedic patients, a fast track in the ED to separate patients by acuity of symptoms, and/or separate units for medical ICU and surgical ICU patients (Litvak, 2005).

Think about the following questions:

- What are the top admission and discharge diagnostic codes for your unit? Your hospital?

- Is your unit or hospital able to meet the needs of these patients?

- Do you have enough case managers and social workers to assist patients with complex medical or socioeconomic needs?

An example of managing this variability is the bariatric population. Although you might not officially have a bariatric program, you still will have patients of size on your unit. Do you have the right equipment to manage them? Bariatric beds, chairs, scales, wheelchairs? How much time is spent working with this patient type or any other for whom you do not have the needed resources to provide efficient care? Besides using staff time to look for resources, it slows the patients' progression through their stay and creates the need for even more staffing and a higher workload.

Remember, use all your resources to help manage the clinical variability of your patients, and schedule your staff to meet these needs! Hospitals can no longer afford to be 8 a.m. to 5 p.m. Monday through Friday operations. Your patient variability demonstrates that. If you need case managers and social workers, respiratory therapists, or a hospitalist to help manage your patient variability, then what are you waiting for? As a nurse manager, you need to build a case that shows better care, better outcomes, and lower costs, even if it means adding (but managing) additional resources.

Patient-Flow Variability

Patient-flow variability is best described by looking at the ED. Although there is some ability to predict variations in peak times when patients come to your ED—Sunday evening, because patients are too ill to wait until Monday to visit the doctor's office, or holiday evenings, when congestive heart failure patients come after a salty holiday dinner—the variability is random. People get sick at different times, for different reasons, and either come in right away or wait to come to your ED.

Patient-flow variability can also refer to patients directly admitted to your unit from the physician's office who are in need of nonelective, urgent admission. Patients who come to your unit for an elective admission are considered artificial variability, which was discussed earlier in this chapter. Many units and hospitals try to manage direct admits, as long as the patient does not just show up on your unit with an order for admission.

How do you manage patient-flow variability? Divide your ED by acuity into a fast track and a regular track. Fast-track patients are low acuity, and regular-track patients are those who are more acutely ill. This way, you have managed the clinical variability in your flow.

Consider the following:

- You may know about all the heart failure and kidney failure patients who come in after a holiday dinner that was not part of their diet, yet do you staff for this seasonal variation?

- Do you have a disaster plan for all types of events that may arise, from flu season to a natural disaster?

- Do you partner and keep in closer contact with those provider offices that may admit more to your unit? Create a process where they contact you at the first sign a patient may need to be admitted to give you more time to plan for a bed and staffing.

Remember: You are trying to manage this type of variability, not eliminate it.

Managing and Staffing for an Influx of ED Patients

In January a few years ago, Arizona, like many states, experienced a high incidence of flu cases. As the emergency director of Yuma Regional Medical Center (YRMC), I was challenged to manage patient flow to handle the additional volume. Although YRMC is a large, 333-bed hospital, it is a rural facility more than 100 miles from any other major hospital, making diversion impossible. The ED was built for a maximum capacity of approximately 125 patients per day, but we were providing care for as many as 300 patients per day.

One creative way we worked to handle the influx in patients was to put a tent in the parking lot to screen and manage the lower-acuity patients, in particular those with flu symptoms. Numerous departments moved quickly to open the temporary tents. Facility maintenance personnel put the tents in place and ensured there was adequate heat. Informatics personnel provided the technology support needed to register and track patients. Dietary personnel installed water coolers and snacks that did not need refrigeration. Equipment, including vital-sign machines, glucose monitors, wheelchairs, and stretchers, was borrowed at night from areas that had a low volume, such as the preoperative care unit, and returned before needed in the morning.

The providers included a rotation of nurse practitioners and physicians. We utilized a variety of staff, including registered nurses, paramedics, and nursing assistants, and designed a patient throughput plan that allowed the appropriate care to occur in a systematic and effective manner. With just a little guidance, staff members were able to create a staffing plan and throughput process to see nearly 100 patients every night for 10 days.

–Teri Wicker, PhD, RN

Professional Variability

Professional variability relates to the way nurses, physicians, and others practice and show up to work. This variability impacts the pace at which patients progress and the number and length of unnecessary delays patients experience (Litvak, 2004). What is considered professional variability?

- Staff skills, motivation, and competing interests (such as mentoring nursing students)

- How staff members organize and manage work (could be artificial as well, depending on why it is organized the way it is)

- Staff illness, medical leave, and disability

- Variations in beliefs on best practice (what is evidence-based practice for one may be different for another)

- Working hours of staff and how staff time off is planned

How does one start to tackle and manage components of professional variability related to staffing and scheduling? Consider the following:

- Review your unit's historical volumes and attempt to match your scheduled staff to your anticipated needs, rather than staffing all days to average.

- Work on improving your nurse retention.

- Know your staff skill mix on each shift. How many new graduate nurses versus experienced nurses do you have? Engage nursing students proactively.

- Assist your staff members in managing their patient care priorities.

- Provide resources and remove barriers that are creating time-consuming workarounds in your unit. Ask staff, "What can I do to make your work easier?"

- The Institute of Medicine states that 90% of practice should be evidence-based by 2020 (National Academy of Sciences, 2009); that's a goal our industry is still working toward in 2024. Where are you? Make all your policies, procedures, and practices evidence-based, and expect your staff to practice evidence-based nursing and medicine.

Patient-flow variability, clinical variability, and professional variability are all types of natural variability. Natural variability cannot be eliminated but can and should be managed to decrease the negative impact on your patient flow and outcomes.

How to Find Your Own Sources of Variability

Now that we have discussed artificial and natural variability, how do we find your sources of variability? The easiest route would be to use (or hire) a process or management engineer to help you with this. The next easiest (and usually free) route is to use a graduate student from your local or state university. The route that will take the most time and energy (although it might be fun if you like these things!) is to do it yourself. We cannot fit all the information you might need into a subsection of a book chapter, but this next section starts you in the right direction.

To begin, you need to determine the sources of your artificial and natural variability. You can impact artificial variation the most, and artificial variation stems from the way you organize your processes, procedures, and environment, usually initially intended to benefit you. But quite often it may actually be counterproductive to quality patient care. How many times have you added to the policy and procedure book? It may be hundreds of pages long. Yet how many times have you taken anything away from it?

Tracers

To do your own high-level analysis, think of a Joint Commission tracer. A *tracer* is a survey methodology in which surveyors choose a patient record and then use it to retrace a patient's movement through the hospital, assessing and evaluating as they go. So, select a patient record, a policy, a procedure, or a workflow, and map it out to assess and evaluate for sources of variation.

Here are some tips to consider while doing a tracer:

- As you perform the tracer and map the process, involve a team of individuals who can collectively help to spot opportunities for improvement and redesign that reduce variation.

- Shadow a patient to collect this data.

- Gather data from a group of patients receiving the same or similar services.

Once you have collected your data, it is time to analyze and evaluate the information. Take the following into consideration while reviewing your data:

- Is there artificial or natural variability?

- If the variability is artificial, what can you do to eliminate it?

- If the variability is natural, how can you manage it?

- Are there patterns to be managed by time of day, day of week, month, and season?

- Is there an impact on your unit's capacity and demand?

- How does this impact other units before or after your unit?

- Is there a mismatch of staff, time off, skill mix, rooms, and/or equipment?

Regardless of whether you use others to assist you in the tracer, you will need to engage others in the solution. As you search for solutions, do keep an open mind. Always ask staff and physicians to help you understand why they may have been doing something a certain way. By approaching the solution with curiosity, you decrease the chance of someone feeling personally attacked, and you will possibly gain a supporter.

Discrete Event Simulation

Another method is *discrete event simulation* (DES), a technique that can create visual models of complex workflow systems (Clissold et al., 2015). A computer model of the process is created using real data. This does require gathering a large amount of data, such as wait times, resource use, and queue sizes, so that simulation of patient-flow processes can be validated against real-world data (Clissold et al., 2015). Expertise in this area would be required. However, you would be very successful in changing your processes correctly the first time based on computer modeling versus multiple changes over time without simulation information.

Making Process Changes

Whether you changed processes based on the tracer or DES method, how do you staff with this in mind? If you have smoothed the artificial variability, your staff resources may be sufficient now to staff to the new and improved (i.e., smaller) peaks and valleys. And if you need additional resources, it will be mainly due to natural variations, in which case you should still have smaller variations in census. Your newly created float pool (see Chapter 3) will be able to help you out there!

This is also where you start with staffing to the new mode (post smoothing) as opposed to the average or mean when you can. How do you figure demand? Go back to Chapter 2 and read about how medians and modes work, and review the example. This will lead you in the right direction. You will need to calculate your own figures for your unit by taking in a year's worth of data if you can, but three years of data is ideal for predictive staffing, removing some of the variability that can occur year-over-year. Unless you have had changes in physician practice affecting volume, you can take the mode each day or week for the last three Septembers and plan your schedule for this September the same. Does your volume demand dip in the summer? Although this adds more complexity, each day might have a different staffing need as you create the schedule. But we already knew it was different day to day. Instead of waiting until today to refigure your staffing needs for today, it will be more effective and safe for your patients to do it ahead of time.

Summary

Here are the key points covered in this chapter:

- Do not just blame your management issues on the idea that your patients are different.

- Peaks in census add unneeded stress to your staff and increase the likelihood of patient death.

- Understand the natural variability that impacts your unit and manage it.

- Understand the artificial variability that impacts your unit and try to eliminate it.

- Find multiple sources of variability using the DES or tracer methodology.

- Involve researchers to help look at your data to co-create a predictive scheduling solution.

References

Aiken, L. H., Clarke, S. P., Sloane, D. M., Sochalski, J. A., & Silber, J. H. (2002). Hospital nurse staffing and patient mortality, nurse burnout, and job dissatisfaction. *Journal of the American Medical Association*, 288(16), 1987–1993. https://doi.org/10.1001/jama.288.16.1987

Asgari, F., & Asgari, S. (2021). Addressing artificial variability in patient flow. *Operations Research for Health Care*, 28, 100288. https://doi.org/10.1016/j.orhc.2021.100288

Bazuin, D. (2010). Patient rooms: A changing scene of healing, creating flexibility for future treatments and technology. *FacilityCare, 15*(6), 22–23.

Clissold, A., Filar, J., Mackay, M., Qin, S., & Ward, D. (2015). *Simulating hospital patient flow for insight and improvement*. Proceedings of the 8th Australasian Workshop on Health Informatics and Knowledge Management.

Litvak, E. (2005). Optimizing patient flow by managing its variability. In Joint Commission Resources, *From front office to front line: Essential issues for health care leaders*, pp. 91–112.

Litvak, E., Buerhaus, P. I., Davidoff, F., Long, M. C., McManus, M. L., & Berwick, D. M. (2005). Managing unnecessary variability in patient demand to reduce nursing stress and improve patient safety. *The Joint Commission Journal on Quality and Patient Safety, 3*(16), 330–338. https://doi.org/10.1016/j.orhc.2021.100288

Litvak, E., Keshavjee, S., Gewertz, B. L., & Fineberg, H. V. (2021). How hospitals can save lives and themselves: Lessons on patient flow from the COVID-19 pandemic. *Annals of Surgery, 274*(1), 37–39. https://doi.org/10.1097/SLA.0000000000004871

McKenna, P., Heslin, S. M., Viccellio, P., Mallon, W. K., Hernandez, C., & Morley, E. J. (2019). Emergency department and hospital crowding: Causes, consequences, and cures. *Clinical and Experimental Emergency Medicine, 6*(3), 189. https://doi.org/10.15441/ceem.18.022

National Academy of Sciences. (2009). *Institute of medicine roundtable on evidence-based medicine.* ncbi.nlm.nih.gov/books/NBK52847/#:~:text=Goal%3A%20By%20the%20year%202020,reflect%20the%20best%20available%20evidence

Target Technology That Improves Staffing and Outcomes

Technology has improved nurses' ability to provide care. In the news, we see examples of robots replacing people, even nurses, scaring us about what might happen in the future. However, think about the glucometer. Up until the first half of the 20th century, clinicians of that time remember the days when the only way to test for diabetes was to sip on a patient's urine to see if it was sweet! We have come to rely on and take for granted some of the technology that has become commonplace in care delivery such as telemetry monitors, MRIs, and computers. For those of us who are old enough, we remember documentation before computers. And now as much as we may dislike documenting on a computer, we dislike downtime more.

In this chapter, we discuss healthcare technology at a high level. There will be some discussion about technology that some hospitals may have, what it means for patient care and nursing, and how it may affect your staffing. There are so many new and emerging technologies that a chapter cannot cover them all, but I point out some principles to be considered for any technology adoption in your unit.

It is important to remember that technology can assist nurses in tasks that enable us to improve patient care. That is a good thing, particularly for the patient, who comes first. However, technology can either decrease or increase a nurse's workload. Additionally, how we incorporate technology may be perceived negatively by the patient, leading to fears of loneliness and loss of autonomy during their hospitalization (Klawunn et al., 2023). All technology should be adopted with a specific goal in mind. All too often organizations want to showcase the latest technology, proven or not, to the community and providers as a way to garner business.

Technology Efficiencies

Staffing and scheduling are impacted by technology. All staffing methods used, whether acuity, workload intensity, ratios, or finance, are impacted by technology. (We talk about staffing methods in Chapter 2.) Some technologies, such as electronic ICU or a remote nurse, may have their own ways to staff and schedule but should not be considered truly independent of the unit or department they serve. As technology advances, improving patient outcomes must be at the forefront of technology integration into practice. The American Nurses Association (ANA) Membership Assembly approved a statement in 2023 that it "supports virtual nursing as a source of support for nurses at the point of care. Virtual nurses should support, but not supplant nursing staff in nursing ratios, matrices, or other measures of staffing levels" (ANA, 2023, p. 7).

As you read this chapter, consider these questions related to your own organization's or unit's technology journey:

- Do you know technology's current impact on your staff and care delivery model?

- Do you need to change your care delivery model to match the technology workflow or vice versa?

- What efficiency will your staff gain through increased use of technology?

- Does technology help nurses spend less time on menial tasks?

- Does it improve patient safety?

- Does it reduce costs?

Consider the following ways that technology can help the nurse:

- Increase efficiency by removing the nurse from the communication chain that does not require their attention

- Help organize work through clinical decision support systems

- Empower the patient to receive education through an interactive system, improving nursing efficiency for other nursing-needed tasks

- Bring information to the point of care

If you are still looking for efficiencies, spend time with the nurses on the floor. Sometimes, nurses have practiced so long a certain way that instead of changing their practice with the new technology, they keep their same practices or have incorporated workarounds as the norm, possibly making care delivery more inefficient. A *workaround* is an informal temporary practice for handling exceptions to normal procedures or workflow (van der Veen et al., 2020). With technology adopted appropriately, such as built-in alignment with nurses' workflows, improvements should be seen, particularly during times of heightened patient acuity.

Although it is unclear whether all technology will positively improve nurses' workload and efficiency, any improvement seen may be offset by the cost of technology. A primary barrier to the implementation of technology is financial. Many organizations have an IT budget for the whole organization that includes a committee and process to review and approve capital and manage equipment *refresh* (the process by which equipment such as computers is replaced regularly). Although the cost of technology may not come directly from your budget, it does lower the overall dollar amount available for the entire organization for other needs.

With the high cost of technology, it must be successfully adopted within your unit's care delivery model. As with any new project, implementation is typically one of the most significant barriers. Those seeking to change practice, mainly to adopt any technology, must recognize that implementation is not an outcome but a continuous, interactive accomplishment (May, 2013). Also, implementation is not a one-time event but rather a bundle of material and cognitive practices (May, 2013) that must evolve to be successful. When a project fails, the implementation process, not the technology, is often the issue. As different technologies are discussed, think about how you would implement, or implement differently, one of them successfully into your unit's or organization's care delivery model.

Artificial Intelligence

Artificial intelligence (AI) "generally applies to computational technologies that emulate mechanisms assisted by human intelligence, such as thought, deep learning, adaptation, engagement, and sensory understanding" (Secinaro et al., 2021, p. 1). Advances in healthcare AI have surged over the last few years thanks to advances in computing power and large amounts of digital data that have been captured (Secinaro et al., 2021). While in early phases of adoption, future uses may support nurses' clinical decision-making in complex care situations or to conduct tasks that are remote (Seibert et al., 2021). Types of decision support include predictive analytics for pressure ulcers, sepsis, and mortality risk.

Appropriate use of AI in nursing practice supports and enhances the core values and ethical obligations of the profession (ANA, 2022). As the nurse manager, ensure policies and procedures regarding AI do not negatively impact the nurse's role. Educating ourselves and direct care nurses about the use and potential benefits and risks of AI is important. This is important so that nurses can be educated and alleviate fears of patients and families who are recipients of AI-assisted care. Organizational or unit/department level policies should never let AI decisions immediately trump nursing decisions. The ANA Code of Ethics clearly states that the nurse is accountable and responsible for nursing practice and the impact on patient care (ANA, 2015).

Consider This

With unlimited possibilities of the use of AI on healthcare, there is widespread fear of the negative impacts. AI raises difficult questions about who makes the call in a health crisis: the human or the machine? In a *Wall Street Journal* article titled "When AI Overrules the Nurses Caring for You," Bannon (2023) provided the potential downfall of such technology when policies limit professional judgment. An oncology nurse was interviewed about an experience she had with a patient who had an AI alarm notify her that her patient had sepsis. The patient had leukemia, and as an experienced oncology nurse, she knew the low white blood cell count that triggered the alarm was most likely due to the cancer, not sepsis. Unfortunately, the policies in place dictated that she start the sepsis protocol, giving the patient a first dose of IV antibiotics while she had to wait for the provider to call back. She was not allowed to call the provider first to discuss this trigger. It was determined later that the patient did not have sepsis and was given medication that the patient did not need. While understanding that timeliness of care is important in managing sepsis, policies must allow for professional judgment and decision-making. One may say, what harm was done? Added expenses and increased resource utilization, among other things.

For AI to positively impact patient care, the ethical challenges must be addressed (World Health Organization [WHO], 2021). WHO has identified six core principles for the ethical use of AI in health (WHO, 2021):

- Protect autonomy.

- Promote human well-being, human safety, and the public interest.

- Ensure transparency, explainability, and intelligibility.

- Foster responsibility and accountability.

- Ensure inclusiveness and equity.

- Promote AI that is responsive and sustainable.

Healthcare organizations and technology companies, as well as nurses, see the value of AI to improve patient care. As with all changes that may impact nurses' work, it is important that direct care nurses are at the table to develop policies and workflows. Incorporate the WHO principles as well as the legal and ethical scope for nurses when integrating AI into practice.

Clinical Decision Support

Clinical decision support (CDS) is defined as a computer system designed to impact clinician decision-making about individual patients at the point in time that these decisions are made (Berner & La Lande, 2007). CDS generally encompasses three steps: acquiring patient data, summarizing data, and suggesting an appropriate course of action (Ramgopal et al., 2023). CDS may include alerts, reminders, order sets, drug-dose calculations, care summary dashboards, and point-of-care information retrieval systems (Ramgopal et al., 2023). The primary purpose of traditional CDS is to assist your staff and physicians at the point of care in determining diagnoses, analyzing patient data, and determining the next steps in care or guiding the next set of interventions.

You may be wondering what the difference is between AI and CDS. In understanding the essential development of CDS, there are two main types: knowledge-based and non-knowledge-based (Berner & LaLande, 2007). A knowledge-based system enables users to edit the knowledge base to keep up with changes in nursing or medicine and then use the data from the knowledge base with the patient's data. A non-knowledge-based system uses machine learning, where the computer learns from experiences and finds patterns in clinical data (Berner & LaLande, 2007). Furthermore, knowledge-based and non-knowledge-based CDS come from algorithms that drive either machine learning (ML) or rules-based expert systems. Traditional CDS may lead to inaccurate or poorly individualized recommendations (Ramgopal et al., 2023), and AI-CDS will lead to better clinical decision. While AI-CDS will lead to better outcomes, not all programs and electronic health records (EHRs) are at the point of incorporating ML within their CDS programs.

Many think of CDS as a system in which the nurses enter data, spit out what they need to do next, and act upon the system's decision. The new way to think of a CDS is as an interactive tool. The CDS assists the nurse, using the nurse's inputs and knowledge with the CDS to help the nurse analyze all the information together. The CDS might give several suggestions and have the nurses choose the actions independently. Additional features of CDS are (Garg et al., 2005):

- Alerts of critical values

- Reminders of overdue preventive health tasks

- Advice for drug prescribing

- Critiques of existing provider orders

- Suggestions for various active care issues

A CDS system can have a positive impact on staffing. Because the system assists your staff members with decisions, they can progress patient care more safely and quickly. A CDS system needs to be considered as you determine your safe staffing needs. The CDS does not replace your nurses or physicians but supports staff members in making complex decisions and enables them to monitor and assess patients more effectively. Usefulness is essential in successfully adopting any technology, including CDS, as any system perceived as not useful is less likely to be adopted (Lopez, Febretti, et al., 2016). Therefore, methods to accelerate the rapid deployment of CDS are needed to improve care (Lopez, Febretti, et al.,

2016). One of the biggest challenges for nurses in using CDS is providing information in such a way that it is valuable and accurate (Lopez, Wilkie, et al., 2016).

Here are some questions to consider when staffing with a CDS system:

- Do you follow a specific nurse-to-patient ratio?

- Can you assess the ability to change the ratio?

- How much time does the CDS save your average nurse?

CDS systems have been shown to improve patient care and may impact nurse staffing. Consider CDS when reviewing workflow, care delivery model, and patient outcomes in determining staffing needs.

Wireless Communication

As with all technology use, security and privacy of the information is of utmost concern. Wireless technology, such as nurse call systems, text messages, and computer documentation systems, is the future and must be incorporated and compliant with the Health Insurance Portability and Accountability Act (HIPAA).

WHO (2007) and The Joint Commission (TJC) have emphasized the importance of communication. Specifically, TJC has long considered communication a top priority, even making it a patient safety goal.

The 2024 Joint Commission National Patient Safety goals include "Improve staff communication [NPSG.02.03.01] Get important test results to the right staff person on time" (TJC, 2024, p. 1). It should be simple, yet the problem is complex with all the ways we communicate with each other in healthcare.

Nurse call systems are not just for nurses but for all staff. They involve wearing an individual wireless device where a staff member or team can be called by name (as opposed to remembering a long list of phone numbers for everyone). Computer documentation systems usually have notification systems that can be turned on to alert and send messages to staff when a lab is complete or when an intervention is needed. And most nurses' favorite: text messages. Many hospital administrators cringed and outlawed text message communication between nurses and physicians because it can violate HIPAA and is not as secure as needed.

However, as younger nurses and clinicians enter the workforce, many default to texting results and orders. Over 85% of physicians and nurses possess smart-phones or tablets, and 60% to 80% of clinical staff exchange text messages related to patient care (Liu et al., 2019). If your organization is considering a secure messaging application, you will need to consider:

- Which clinical processes to improve
- How to archive text messages
- How to manage mobile devices
- How to dictate a bring-your-own-device policy.
- How to maintain wi-fi architecture

Organizations should not allow staff to text patient information without a secure messaging application. By providing a HIPAA-compliant communication platform, organizations can improve clinical collaboration and workflow (Liu et al., 2019).

Consider This

Think about a wireless badge system. You will decrease overhead pages significantly, decrease the time other staff spends looking for someone, and decrease mass management of cellphones.

In addition to the expense of purchasing technology, such as a wireless nurse-call system, hospitals' infrastructure may not support it. As technology changes, the demand for power and bandwidth changes as well. Hospitals must add more lines or completely replace old wiring for wireless technology to work.

Nonetheless, here are the positive impacts of wireless communication on staffing, which may outweigh the costs associated with implementing such a system:

- Health unit secretaries spend less time "calling people."
- Information and alerts can be communicated in real time.
- Clinicians can act sooner due to shorter wait times for information.
- Length of stay is reduced due to minimized delays in care.

Wireless communication can improve communication among caregivers and facilitate safe patient care. In the last several years, wireless communication has gained traction in every aspect of healthcare, including requesting appointments, refilling medications, and even paying bills. Consider this technology for your unit, remembering to consider patient safety, nurse efficiency, communication, and budget.

Electronic Health Records

An EHR, or electronic medical record (EMR), is more than a paper version of the patient's hospital chart. With the varied implementation and now re-implementation of EHRs, nurses have given the EHR a mixed review. Some staff members complain that it causes more work, primarily if they work in a paper and electronic health record hybrid.

Documentation is important as it allows nurses to note the nursing process, including interventions and outcomes. Researchers have noted that documentation completeness was associated with improved patient outcomes and resource utilization in patients transferred between hospitals (Usher et al., 2016). Yet, nurses spend as much as 25% to 41% of their time on documentation (De Groot et al., 2022). This amount of time, while spent on an important task, is perceived negatively on the overall workload of nurses. It is important regardless of the EHR to continue to improve the user-friendliness, improve the intercommunicability of different electronic systems, and further integrate clinical documentation so that time spent documenting can be decreased and more time spent on direct patient care activities (De Groot et al., 2022).

Even with mixed reviews from staff and patients, a national mandate is tied to payment to adopt EHR systems in all hospitals and provider clinics. The American Recovery and Reinvestment Act (ARRA) of 2009, also known affectionately as the Stimulus or the Recovery Act, was in response to the recession, and its primary purpose was to save and create jobs. Secondarily, it was to invest in infrastructure and health, among other things. As of 2019, 95% of hospitals had adopted an EHR (Parasrampuria & Henry, 2019).

ARRA included enacting the Health Information Technology for Economic and Clinical Health Act, also known as the HITECH Act. Before the Affordable Care Act of 2010, this act was considered the most critical piece of healthcare legislation in 30 years. The point of the act is not just to put in an EHR but to use it meaningfully by having providers and healthcare staff achieve significant improvements in care. The ARRA timeline had, and continues to have, many requirements and penalties for missing those requirements. One penalty is that hospitals that begin certified EHR use after 2015 are not eligible for incentive payments. While the focus of ARRA has been on hospitals and physician practices, further research is needed to fully understand the complexities of the EHR in all settings (Carrington et al., 2016), as care is increasingly occurring outside the hospital setting. As of 2017, 94% of hospitals used their EHR data to perform hospital processes that inform clinical practice (Parasrampuria & Henry, 2019). EHR data is most commonly used by hospitals to support quality improvement (82%), monitor patient safety (81%), and measure organization performance (77%; Parasrampuria & Henry, 2019).

TIP

For a successful adoption, role-modeling appropriate use of the EHR while caring for the patient is critical. Even the most expert nurse who has worked 10, 20, or 30 years in a paper record is a novice nurse in the EHR. On the other hand, a younger nurse steeped in technology may not fully appreciate HIPAA concerns. Learn the EHR yourself if you haven't used it, and demonstrate how they can merge their documentation with their practice in real time to become expert nurses in the EHR.

Staffing for a Go-Live

The answer to how to staff for a go-live may be the holy grail of EHR implementations or reimplementation. With all the time and effort placed into implementing an EHR, it is surprising today that so many organizations have decided to change vendors completely and go through this process yet again. Partner with the new EHR vendor for examples from other go-lives related to best practices. The vendor wants a positive implementation as do you!

Consider these costs and staffing points when planning for go-live:

- What is the needed super user to staff ratio?

- How much time is needed for classroom education?

- Are there different classes and lengths of education by staff position?

- How long do the super users themselves train prior to going live?

- How much time will the super users need for ongoing system education?

- How long is the recommended time to have super users out of the count to assist staff at go-live?

- Is this coming from your budget, or is there a central budget for these costs?

- What is the average time for staff to become comfortable with the EHR?

- For your per diem or part-time staff members, how will you ensure their education and competency?

- Who will assess ongoing competency and appropriate use of the system?

- Do you get to alter productivity targets for the go-live?

Budget Considerations for Staffing a Go-live

I once was in charge of the clinical operations aspect of go-live for our new hospital registration, scheduling, and bed board (this was the first phase of the rollout for our new EMR). The company stated that the ratio of super users to end users was 1:8. When company employees started to work with our IT department, they considered all unit staff as super users (and noted that the cost was coming out of the individual unit's budget). If this plan had gone forward, it would have been a very pricey and over-staffed go-live. Not every staff RN needed access to the first phase EMR components. Instead, we designated super users for those who needed it, such as the charge nurses, unit secretaries, and case managers, which was more cost-effective. Instead of having multiple super users scheduled per floor, we needed only one super user per several floors.

–Jennifer Mensik-Kennedy, PhD, RN, NEA-BC, FAAN

Implementing or changing your EHR is a resource-intensive process and can significantly impact staffing levels during the learning curve. Understand the impact of a go-live on your unit and your staff to ensure the best utilization of super users and support to minimize costs to your unit and organization.

Electronic Medication Administration With Barcoding

There have been many system redesigns around medication administration. Dedicated medication nurses and self-directed education do not reduce medica-tion errors (Greengold et al., 2003; Schneider et al., 2006). A literature review on barcode-assisted medication administration systems showed reduced medication error rates (Hassink et al., 2012). The handheld scanner used with barcoding-assisted medication administration quickly identifies the five rights of medication administration once the medication is scanned and the patient's identification band is scanned. Longtime nurses may remember learning, as well as teaching, medication administration, and the process was supposed to happen three times with the old-fashioned, nonelectronic method: first time in reviewing the order/medication sheet, second while pulling out the medication, and third and final during the actual administration. Then, we graduated from nursing school and needed to find ways to work more quickly. Plus, after a while with medication administration, we felt like experts and, knowingly or not, shortened the five rights processes at those three critical points.

Barcoding does reduce medication errors in hospitals, specifically preventing targeted wrong dose, wrong drug, wrong patient, unauthorized drug, and wrong route errors (Hutton et al., 2021).

However, it is important to note that even with technology, processes are skipped, or barcoding may not be available in all areas. Fatal medication errors still occur today despite technology. Technology doesn't replace critical thinking.

Here are the implications of electronic medication administration for staffing:

- What is the impact of barcoding and timely medication administration if you have a functional, team, or primary care delivery model?

- Are there enough scanners for each nurse? Or do you make nurses share? Knowing that the Centers for Medicare & Medicaid Services has requirements for timely passing of medications, and most meds are scheduled simultaneously, you will be frustrating staff members and decreasing their productivity if they do not have individual scanners.

- With the scanners, are the docking stations located centrally, or are they placed around the unit to decrease the time your staff spends looking for scanners?

- Do all departments use bar scanners? Do you use them in fast-moving and time-sensitive departments like the ED and ICU? If so, do you need more staff to assist in passing medications?

- If you are going live, will you need to staff up to support the learning curve?

Medication administration technology can improve patient safety and outcomes. Staff members may believe this technology negatively impacts their efficiency; therefore, it is important for the manager to understand how the preceding factors may impact your unit and increase workloads.

Remote Monitoring/Telehealth

When we think of remote surveillance, we tend to think of telehealth in the community. However, think of this as telehealth for the acute care setting. Various remote surveillance models exist, including simple video monitoring or the much more complex electronic, or *tele*, ICU. As technology progresses, lengths of stay become shorter, reimbursement dwindles, and it becomes increasingly important to incorporate technology into our care delivery models to support patient care and improve outcomes. Remote or tele monitoring can occur in many settings; however, it is most often used in cardiovascular, neurology, pulmonary, obstetrics, and intensive care areas. Research of telehealth in these areas has shown that while it can decrease mortality rates in these areas, telehealth hasn't increased mortality rates (Snoswell et al., 2023).

Continuous Video Monitoring

Continuous video monitoring (CVM) at a basic level is just that: monitoring a patient through a video camera and a television. This level of technology usually does not include predictive analytics. CVM should be considered a bridge for nurses to enhance patient safety and when sitters may not be an option (Abbe & O'Keeffe, 2021). Technology is not a replacement for RNs, and it cannot be used with every patient. It can, when applied appropriately, be used to successfully augment the oversight of a specific patient to improve care while reducing care costs. Incorporation of CVM into a unit's care delivery should always include the direct care nurse's perspective. Table 7.1 includes the CVM considerations for use on pediatric and adult patients (Abbe & O'Keeffe, 2021).

TABLE 7.1   CVM CONSIDERATIONS FOR USE ON PEDIATRIC AND ADULT PATIENTS

Inclusion Criteria	Exclusion Criteria
Drug/alcohol withdrawal	Behavioral restraints
Delirium	Seclusion
Restfulness	High-risk suicide
Confusion (acute or chronic)	Failure of a two-hour trial period on camera
Safety restraints	All phases of eating disorder during mealtimes (pediatric only)
Medication device protection	
Elopement risk	
General safety concerns	
Fall prevention	
Eating disorders	
Low/moderate suicide risk	

Electronic Intensive Care

The tele-ICU is a network of audiovisual and computer systems that provides the basis for an interprofessional care model for critically ill patients. Tele-ICU service is not designed to replace local services but to augment care through leveraging resources and standardizing processes. Tele-intensive care combines video monitoring, CDS, and expert physicians and RNs who continuously act as an additional support layer for intensive care patients in the hospital.

Tele-intensive care has a profound impact on staffing and scheduling—not only for the organization using this technology through improved utilization of critical care services but also for the quality of patient care on units that are being monitored such as decreased mortality rates (Fusaro et al., 2019). Sharing critical care resources is beneficial in an urban setting, and rural and Critical Access Hospitals that utilize tele-ICU gain increased expertise from experienced intensive-care physicians and nurses who work in much larger critical care units in addition to the risk prediction algorithms, smart alarm systems, and machine learning tools the technology provides (Khurrum et al., 2021). Novice nurses will have more around-the-clock support from expert ICU nurses, particularly at night when there always seem to be more novice nurses and fewer resources.

While tele-ICU has been widely adopted, research is still needed to compare the various models and approaches taken across different organizations to determine best practices with this technology (Subramanian et al., 2020). One study using a mobile platform with a rapid response team noted cost avoidance from unnecessary ICU transfers that supported a return on investment of up to $1.66 for every $1.00 invested in IT support (Pappas et al., 2016).

Electronic intensive care is an intensivist-led team located separately from an office's hospital and inpatient ICU beds. It may be considered the "hub" like an air-traffic control tower. Electronic ICU does not house patients or replace the hospital ICU, physicians, RNs, or staff but supplements the care given in this setting. The electronic ICU is usually staffed with board-certified intensivists, acute care nurse practitioners, and experienced critical care nurses. The hub has two-way voice, video, and data technology for the staff to "take care of" the ICU patients remotely. The physicians and nurses execute predefined plans or intervene in emergencies when a patient's attending physician is not in the ICU.

Typical staffing ratios are as follows for the different clinicians in the electronic ICU hub:

- One tele-intensivist ratio is about 50–100 (Canfield et al., 2022).

- Two to three eRN to 50–100 beds (Canfield et al., 2022)

- One clerical assistant to 50–125 patients (Goran, 2010)

An electronic ICU has the following components:

- **Smart alerts:** Patient information, such as physiologic and laboratory data, flows from the bedside medical record into the electronic ICU software, where algorithms look for trends in data and alert the electronic ICU staff. Care interventions occur earlier because monitored patient information is processed faster and the intensivist or RN can intervene earlier, usually stopping an adverse event. Software prompts indicate when a patient is straying "out of bounds" (e.g., early sepsis), enabling the electronic ICU physician to intervene, often precluding an adverse event.

- **Clinical documentation:** Some electronic ICU software has an EHR component that may be used at the bedside and in the hub. Interfaces are built to send data seamlessly between two different systems.

- **Evidence-based practice:** Standards of care are maintained and often improved as clinical data and best practices are built into the system for clinician triggers.

- **Outcomes:** Clinical outcomes, resource utilization, and operational efficiency are tied to the Agency for Healthcare Research and Quality recommendations and are regularly tracked with the electronic ICU programs' reporting solutions. Daily management tools enable real-time, patient-specific analysis for compliance with best practices. Ad hoc queries can be customized to facilitate ongoing research.

There are some considerations for staffing your patient side of the ICU or the electronic ICU hub, including the following:

- Consider hiring only experienced ICU nurses. It is preferable that an RN's minimum years of experience in the electronic ICU hub is 10 years in critical care, preferably 15 years.

- With this level of expert ICU nurses, more novice nurses at the bedside have another resource and mentor/preceptor to enhance their learning, provide safer care, and answer questions or address concerns.

- Older nurses enjoy the electronic ICU role, allowing them to maintain their knowledge and productivity. RNs are very involved with patient care while not having to stand 12 hours daily.

- Due to the rapid rise in electronic ICUs, certification is now available to RNs who work in this setting.

- Although an electronic ICU does not replace minimum staffing levels or RNs at the bedside, it may positively affect the 1:1 RN-to-patient ratio at the bedside in the ICU, allowing them to expand to a 1 RN-to-2 ICU patient ratio more often based on patient condition. With the advances in technology, surveillance, and the ability of the electronic ICU staff, the bedside RN has more than just a second set of eyes.

- Initial barriers to an electronic ICU with staff include the reluctance to work with the electronic ICU RNs, such as the feeling that they are "big brother watching."

Tele-intensive care has demonstrated improved patient outcomes and decreased lengths of stay. There are multiple implications for effective and efficient nurse staffing in the hub and on the unit for nursing that need to be assessed by the nurse manager.

Summary

Here are the key points covered in this chapter:

- Implementation of technology should always include and involve direct care nurses who are end users.

- Virtual nurses should support but not supplant nursing staff.

- CDS systems can improve efficiencies.

- Electronic ICUs can reduce mortality and length of stay.

- Electronic ICUs can impact workload and 1:1 nurse-to-patient needs at the bedside.

- Novice nurses will have more around-the-clock support from expert ICU nurses, particularly at night when there always seem to be more novice nurses and fewer resources.

References

Abbe, J. R., & O'Keeffe, C. (2021). Continuous video monitoring: Implementation strategies for safe patient care and identified best practices. *Journal of Nursing Care Quality, 36*(2), 137.

American Nurses Association. (2015). *Code of ethics for nurses with interpretive statements: Development, interpretation, and application* (2nd ed.). Author.

American Nurses Association. (2022). *The ethical use of artificial intelligence in nursing practice.* https://www.nursingworld.org/~48f653/globalassets/practiceandpolicy/nursing-excellence/ana-position-statements/the-ethical-use-of-artificial-intelligence-in-nursing-practice_bod-approved-12_20_22.pdf

American Nurses Association. (2023). *Summary of the 2023 annual meeting of the ANA Membership Assembly.* https://www.nursingworld.org/~4a7374/globalassets/ana leadership--governance/ma/2023-ma-summary.pdf

Bannon, L. (2023, June 15). When AI overrules the nurses caring for you. *Wall Street Journal.* https://www.wsj.com/articles/ai-medical-diagnosis-nurses-f881b0fe

Berner, E., & La Lande, T. (2007). *Clinical decision support systems: Theory and practice.* Springer.

Canfield, C., Perez-Protto, S., Siuba, M., Hata, S., & Udeh, C. (2022). Beyond the nuts and bolts: Tele-critical care patients, workflows, and activity patterns. *Telemedicine and e-Health, 28*(1). https://doi.org/10.1089/tmj.2020.0452

Carrington, J. M., Tiase, V., Estrada, N., Shea, K. D., Finley, B. A., Nibbelink, C., Shea, K. D., Dudding, K. M., Finley, B. A., Nibbelink, C., Rasmussen, R. J., & Roberts, M. L. (2016). Nursing informatics research and emerging trends in 2015. *CIN: Computers, Informatics, Nursing, 34*(7), 284–286. https://doi.org/10.1097/CIN.0000000000000278

De Groot, K., De Veer, A. J. E., Munster, A. M., Francke, A. L., & Paans, W. (2022). Nursing documentation and its relationship with perceived nursing workload: A mixed-methods study among community nurses. *BMC Nursing, 21*, 34. https://doi.org/10.1186/s12912-022-00811-7

Fusaro, M. V., Becker, C., & Scurlock, C. (2019). Evaluating tele-ICU implementation based on observed and predicted ICU mortality: A systematic review and meta-analysis. *Critical Care Medicine, 47*(4), 501–507. https://doi.org/10.1097/CCM.0000000000003627

Garg, A. X., Adhikari, N. K. J., McDonald, H., Rosas-Arellano, M. P., Devereaux, P. J., Beyene, J., Sam, J., & Haynes, R. B. (2005). Effects of computerized clinical decision support systems on practitioner performance and patient outcomes: A systematic review. *Journal of the American Medical Association, 293*(10), 1223–1238. https://doi.org/10.1001/jama.293.10.1223

Goran, S. F. (2010). A second set of eyes: An introduction to tele-ICU. *Critical Care Nurse, 30*(4), 46–55. https://doi.org/10.4037/ccn2010283

Greengold, N. L., Shane, R., Schneider, P., Flynn, E., Elashoff, J., Hoying, C. L., Barker, K., & Bolton, L. B. (2003). The impact of dedicated medication nurses on the medication administration error rate: A randomized controlled trial. *Archives of Internal Medicine, 163*(19), 2359–2367. https://doi.org/10.1001/archinte.163.19.2359

Hassink, J. J. M., Jansen, M. M. P. M., & Helmons, P. J. (2012). Effects of bar-code-assisted medication administration (BCMA) on frequency, type and severity of medication administration errors: A review of the literature. *European Journal of Hospital Pharmacy-Science and Practice, 19,* 489–494.

Hutton, K., Ding, Q., & Wellman, G. (2021). The effects of bar-coding technology on medication errors: A systematic literature review. *Journal of Patient Safety, 17*(3), e192–e206. https://doi.org/10.1097/PTS.0000000000000366

The Joint Commission. (2024). *2024 Hospital National Patient Safety Goals.* https://www.jointcommission.org/-/media/tjc/documents/standards/national-patient-safety-goals/2024/hap-npsg-simple-2024-v2.pdf

Khurrum, M., Asmar, S., & Joseph, B. (2021). Telemedicine in the ICU: Innovation in the critical care process. *Journal of Intensive Care Medicine, 36*(12), 1377–1384. https://doi.org/10.1177/0885066620968518

Klawunn, R., Albrecht, U.-V., & Dierks, M.-L. (2023). Expectations of new technologies in nursing care among hospital patients in Germany–An interview study. *Frontiers in Psychology, 14*(14), 1227852. https://doi.org/10.3389/fpsyg.2023.1227852

Liu, X., Sutton, P. R., McKenna, R., Sinanan, M. N., Fellner, B. J., Leu, M. G., & Ewell, C. (2019). Evaluation of secure messaging applications for a health care system: A case study. *Applied Clinical Informatics, 10*(1), 140–150. https://doi.org/10.1055/s-0039-1678607

Lopez, K. D., Febretti, A., Stifter, J., Johnson, A., Wilkie, D. J., & Keenan, G. (2016). Toward a more robust and efficient usability testing method of clinical decision support for nurses derived from nursing electronic health record data. *International Journal of Nursing Knowledge, 28*(4), 211–218. https://doi.org/10.1111/2047-3095.12146

Lopez, K. D., Wilkie, D. J., Yao, Y., Sousa, V., Febretti, A., Stifter, J., Johnson, A., & Keenan, G. M. (2016). Nurses' numeracy and graphical literacy: Informing studies of clinical decision support interfaces. *Journal of Nursing Care Quality, 31*(2), 124–130. https://doi.org/10.1097/NCQ.0000000000000149

May, C. (2013). Towards a general theory of implementation. *Implementation Science, 8*(18), 1–14. https://doi.org/10.1186/1748-5908-8-18

Pappas, P., Tirelli, L., Shaffer, J., & Gettings, S. (2016). Projecting critical care beyond ICU: An analysis of tele ICU support for rapid response teams. *Telemedicine and e-Health, 22*(6), 529–533. https://doi.org/10.1089/tmj.2015.0098

Parasrampuria, S., & Henry, J. (2019, April). *Hospitals' use of electronic health records data, 2015–2017.* ONC data brief no. 46. Office of the National Coordinator for Health Information Technology.

Ramgopal, S., Sanchez-Pinto, L. N., Horvat, C. M., Carroll, M. S., Luo, Y., & Florin, T. A. (2023). Artificial intelligence-based clinical decision support in pediatrics. *Pediatric Research, 93,* 334–341. https://doi.org/10.1038/s41390-022-02226-1

Schneider, P. J., Pedersen, C. A., Montanya, K. R., Curran, C. R., Harpe, S. E., Bohenek, W., Perrato, B., Swaim, T. J., & Wellman, K. E. (2006). Improving the safety of medication administration using an interactive CD-ROM program. *American Journal of Health-System Pharmacy, 63*(1), 59–64. https://doi.org/10.2146/ajhp040609

Secinaro, S., Calandra, D., Secinaro, A., Muthurangu, V., & Biancone, P. (2021). The role of artificial intelligence in healthcare: A structured literature review. *BMC Medical Informatics and Decision Making, 21*(1), 125. https://doi.org/10.1186/s12911-021-01488-9

Seibert, K., Domhoff, D., Bruch, D., Schulte-Althoff, M., Fürstenau, D., Biessmann, F., & Wolf-Ostermann, K. (2021). Application scenarios for artificial intelligence in nursing care: Rapid review. *Journal of Medical Internet Research, 23*(11), e26522.

Snoswell, C. L., Stringer, H., Taylor, M. L., Caffery, L. J., & Smith, A. C. (2023). An overview of the effect of telehealth on mortality: A systematic review of meta-analyses. *Journal of Telemedicine and Telecare, 29*(9), 659–668. https://doi.org/10.1177/1357633X211023700

Subramanian, S., Pamplin, J. C., Hravnak, M., Hielsberg, C., Riker, R., Rincon, F., Laudanski, K., Adzhigirey, L. A., Moughrabieh, M. A., Winterbottom, F. A., & Herasevich, V. (2020). Tele-critical care: An update from the society of critical care medicine tele-ICU committee. *Critical Care Medicine, 48*(4), 553–561.

Usher, M. G., Fanning, C., Wu, D., Balonze, K., Kim, D., Parikh, A., & Herrigel, D. (2016). Information handoff and outcomes of critically ill patients transferred between hospitals. *Journal of Critical Care, 10*(36), 240–245. https://doi.org/10.1016/j.jcrc.2016.08.006

van der Veen, W., Taxis, K., Wouters, H., Vermeulen, H., Bates, D. W., van den Bemt, P. M. L. A., & BCMA Study Group. (2020). Factors associated with workarounds in barcode-assisted medication administration in hospitals. *Journal of Clinical Nursing, 29*(13–14), 2239–2250. https://doi.org/10.1111/jocn.15217

WHO Collaborating Centre for Patient Safety Solutions. (2007, May). Communication during patient hand-overs. *Patient Safety Solutions, 1*(3). https://cdn.who.int/media/docs/default-source/patient-safety/patient-safety-solutions/ps-solution3-communication-during-patient-handovers.pdf

World Health Organization. (2021). *Ethics and governance of artificial intelligence for health: WHO guidance.* https://www.who.int/publications/i/item/9789240029200

CHAPTER

8

Pulling Your Data Together

We have all heard at one point in our careers a colleague say things such as, "That is not the way we do things here," or, "We've tried that before," implying it won't work now. This can be disheartening, especially when you know change needs to occur, and you are making the effort to lead it. So, if you encounter this, do not be dismayed. A mentor once said, "A good idea at the wrong time is a bad idea." So, what did not work then may work now. People change (literally and figuratively), times change, organizations change. The issue just might have been timing. Do not hesitate to point that out. That was then, and this is now. Things are different, and it is worth another try.

This chapter reviews the key components affecting your schedule and scheduling process and provides helpful hints and potential solutions. We also review direct, nondirect, indirect, productive, and nonproductive time and show you how to calculate these numbers.

Where Do You Go From Here?

Where do you go from here? If you are new to staffing and scheduling, this can be overwhelming. Maybe you are taking over a unit or department that is well organized and staffed. But maybe you were selected to be the person to fix a problem. When you have a job that will require a lot of work, it is helpful to think about a quote attributed to Robert H. Lauer: "Nothing worthwhile ever happens quickly and easily. You achieve only as you are determined to achieve ... and as you keep at it until you have achieved."

So, where do you start and how do you start? Let's start with the nursing process as the guide: Assessment, Diagnosis, Planning, Intervention, and Evaluation. First, you must assess your unit's and organization's policies, processes, procedures, and guidelines as well as outcomes. What and where is your actual starting point? Then, diagnose the issues so you can start planning! Interventions will be incorporating what you have learned in this book to build and explain your ideal staffing and care delivery model. And of course, evaluate. Understand your unit's outcomes on the unit level, as well as employee and patient outcomes.

In your assessment, include vital unit-specific measures with real-time data so that you can make the best—and predictive—staffing and scheduling decisions. By now, you should understand your base staffing needs and what positions you may need, so how do you avoid holes in the schedule and daily staffing?

Earlier in Chapter 3, we discussed a float pool, but remember, sometimes you may need to rely on that to fill your holes. Roster management, or position control, is a great way to organize your human resources. It will help you understand your full-time equivalent (FTE) needs at a glance, how many positions are filled and by whom, who is on orientation, and what hiring you still need to do. This document is an essential component that makes workforce planning more manageable and organized. For an example of a position control sheet, see Chapter 11.

A confusing point in your budget may be that you have two distinct numbers for employees: employees as a number of actual people and employees added together to determine the number of FTEs you have. Remember, the number of staff you have is usually greater than your total FTE number. This is where your roster management becomes very helpful. This sheet (sometimes an Excel work-sheet) will note the names of your staff members and their FTEs as well as their assigned shift (i.e., day, night). A full-time, 40-hour-a-week employee is a 1.0 FTE. An RN who is assigned three 12-hour shifts weekly is a 0.9 FTE; an RN who works two 12-hour shifts is a 0.6 FTE. Every four hours an employee was not hired to work in a week equals a 0.1 decrease in the FTE status. As you plan for education and other events, it is essential to note whether you consider your staff numbers by total FTEs or physical bodies.

TIP

Remember that not all hours worked are in direct, hands-on patient care. Assume that 75% to 85% of potential hours are productive (due to vacation, sick time, education, etc.). Each full-time staff RN who is 85% productive results in an annual rate of 1,768 hours of direct patient care.

In your current scheduling and staffing process, as well as on your position control sheet, you need to consider how you plan for the following:

- Sick time

- Overtime

- Agency/traveler use

- Unit turnover rate (transfers and resignations)

- Pregnancies and maternity leave

- FMLA (Family and Medical Leave Act)/LOA (leave of absence)

- Budgeted FTEs

- Current vacancies

- Time to hire (from resignation letter to start date of replacement RNs)

- Time your replacement RNs start until they complete orientation

- Staff competence, education, and certification levels
- Maximum scheduled shifts in a row

Day and shift changes in staffing and needs based on these issues create a lot of work, and maybe even chaos, for you and your staff. Planning and spending adequate time appropriately preparing the schedule takes time. One study noted that charge nurses reported spending up to 90% of a shift resolving intrashift staffing issues (Wilson et al., 2011). What do you want your charge nurses to do? There are many other things your charge nurses can be doing to gain management and leadership skills rather than dealing with the result of a bad schedule and poor staffing.

Consider This

If your workforce planning and schedules are solely based on last year's staffing patterns and census, you are setting yourself up for failure. How many days or months last year were there staffing issues? Scheduling problems and budget issues? So, knowing that, why would you still use last year's data to project next year's needs? You have to stop and be the one to clean up the data!

TIP

If you staff to your midnight average daily census (ADC) and find that you do not have the staff needed to reflect the churn in your day, think about using this modified version of an ADC. Take your midnight ADC and add half a "point" to each discharge you had in the previous 24 hours. So, if your midnight ADC is 24, and you had six discharges, your modified ADC is 27 [24 + (6 x 0.5)]. You can now determine your needed FTEs based on this modified ADC that better reflects your unit's needs.

Unit Assessment

To start your unit assessment, read your unit's and organization's policies and procedures on staffing, scheduling, and time off. Also, be sure to have your completed roster management sheet in front of you (see Chapter 11 if you still need to create one). This document will give you an understanding of what staff you have, how many FTEs that equals, and how your position control sheet compares to your budget. From here, you can start to understand what influences your staffing.

> **TIP**
>
> *Just because your budget or position control document says something now does not mean it is the correct number. You will need to do some adjusting to get it right. Remember, you need to update all this data quarterly. Things change—technology changes, physicians switch hospitals and referral patterns, and even your patients may change acuity. Also, try the modified ADC.*

As with everything you do, always find out your organization's policy, definitions, and formulas. See Chapter 2 in case you need a refresher. The following section reviews additional calculations related to productive and nonproductive time.

Workload Measurement

Workload measurement means what it says: It is the measurement of work requirements. It can also be referred to as *acuity and intensity*. This can include the time, skills, and knowledge needed to perform specific interventions within various categories or domains of care (Scherb & Weydt, 2009). It should also include nursing judgment. These domains are typically informed using a nursing classification or standardized language system. These methods of determining workload are very labor-intensive. Acuity software systems can do this for you, at a cost, of course. Some organizations have chosen to build their own systems that take into consideration work intensity. Examples of standardized language systems that may be used in an acuity software program include:

- Nursing Interventions Classification (NIC)

- Nursing Outcomes Classification (NOC)

- North American Nursing Diagnosis Association International (NANDA-I)

- Systematized Nomenclature of Medicine—Clinical Terms (SNOMED CT)

- Omaha System

Workload measurement has also been used in relationship to diagnosis-related groups (DRGs) or case mix index (CMI). The trouble with using DRGs is that they are a medical diagnosis, and the amount of nursing work between two patients with a DRG of hysterectomy may be vastly different. The CMI has the same issue. The CMI is the average DRG weight for all Medicare volumes. Although nursing care does depend partly on the medical diagnosis, it does not measure the nursing components of care.

You need to know whether your organization uses any workload measurement already; if not, determine this using your unit's average CMI. The best solution is to buy acuity-based staffing software that determines your acuity.

Workload Calculations

To determine workload, you need to measure your workload, whatever that may be. As mentioned previously, you might use DRG or CMI. Once your workload is quantified into an average number, you can determine the total number of FTEs you need based on your acuity instead of solely on historical staffing or finance data. Remember, we review how to determine your hours per patient day (HPPD) in Chapter 2.

Here is how to calculate FTEs for a unit based on acuity (Dugan Claudio, 2004):

1. Direct hours
   Acuity/workload measure x target hours = direct care HPPD

2. Nondirect hours
   Nondirect FTEs for the unit x 40 hours / 168 = nondirect HPPD

3. Total HPPD
   Direct HPPD + nondirect HPPD = total HPPD

4. FTEs
   Total HPPD x ADC x 365 / 2,080 hours per 1.0 FTE = total FTEs

NOTE

Target hours should be, in part, based on professional standards. Example: Your professional organization states that 5.0 hours of nursing care per patient per day should be required. What is the difference here? Remember, considering the professional standard, we are figuring out HPPD based on acuity.

So now you have figured out your FTE need based on workload. Again, as with your ADC, use that number here if you can use the modified ADC (the one that considers churn with points for discharge). Remember that this is only the workload calculation to determine the FTEs needed if they all showed up to work each day, never got sick, never went on vacation, and you have no turnover.

"Nonproductive" Time

So, at this point you have figured out or know how to figure out how many FTEs you need for quality staffing and scheduling based on your patients' needs. However, there are more steps! The preceding number assumes that your nurses never take time off. This downtime might be called something different at your organization, such as *benefit replacement* or *allowance time*, but it is typically considered *nonproductive*. This nonproductive time bucket includes everything from breaks and meals, to inservices, education, staff development, and more. This does not sound nonproductive at all! Why do we call nonproductive time, non-productive time? This phrasing is an insult to nurses and the profession. With our physician colleagues, their "non" productive time is called administrative time. Of course physician administrative time includes documentation and paperwork. Can you imagine if we moved the time nurses spent documenting into administrative time! Finance and administration might start to consider improving the EHRs.

It is by far time that we use the same language for nurses. Words matter. The activities completed during administrative time by nurses have a positive impact on patients.

To make the appropriate adjustments and hire sufficient staff to cover leave of all kinds, consider a 22% allowance (Summers, 2016). However, this may range between 15% and 25%. Your organization may have its number, so ask first.

Here is an example of how to calculate nonproductive time:

> Take the prior FTE count from the calculation before (results of step 4) x 1.22.

This equals the total number of FTEs for your schedule, including coverage of vacation, sick time, and other types of leave.

Remember, your organization's ratio may differ from 1.22, which is the allowance recommended by the ICN. Also, know whether your organization includes nondirect time in your organization's nonproductive time. You want to avoid including nondirect time twice in your productive and nonproductive numbers.

Staffing for Direct, Indirect, and Nondirect Time

Some organizations further break out and manage direct, indirect, and nondirect time. There may be overlap between these and productive and nonproductive time. *Direct time* is nursing care that directly involves the patient (i.e. physical assessment, education). *Indirect time* is nursing activities on behalf of the patient but not directly with the patient (i.e. care conference, documentation). *Indirect time* also refers to the time spent by staff members who do not flex, such as unit clerks, charge nurses, and support staff. *Nondirect time* consists of activities conducted not on behalf of an individual patient directly or indirectly (i.e. meetings, education); it is sometimes referred to as *nonproductive time*.

Sit down and talk with your finance liaison to understand how your organization defines and manages these definitions. Also make sure you know where to find these reports and how to interpret the data.

With budget and staffing, you do have the ability to plan for various buckets of time as well as trending past years usages to project future time needs such as historical FMLA, meeting and education times, as well as orientations. You can control and have flexibility with these items.

It is vital to benchmark these numbers as well. The Labor Management Institute (2009) provides a benchmark for indirect hours by service line (see Table 8.1).

TABLE 8.1   INDIRECT HOURS BENCHMARK BY SERVICE LINE

Service Line	Percentage of Indirect Hours
Critical care	13.2%
Intermediate care and specialty units	15.9%
General medical-surgical	11.4%
Women's and children's	14.1%
Perioperative services	15.5%
Emergency department and other units	20.1%
Behavioral health and skilled nursing	18.6%

The following formulas assist you in determining how your budget and staffing numbers go together and what they mean to your budget:

Total productive time (hours) includes direct time + nondirect time

Total productive time + indirect time + nonproductive time = the total dollars needed in your budget

The best way to figure out these numbers is to know your total budget and benchmark it against other databases, hospitals, and like units to determine what you want to set as a budget for indirect time and nondirect time.

Frontline Leadership Schedules

Frontline leaders are usually the charge nurses. You might have charge nurses in or out of the count, meaning they may or may not take patients based on your unit's needs. If you have dedicated charge nurses who do not take patients unless a critical need occurs on the unit, consider how you schedule them related to time. Does your charge nurse work 12-hour shifts if your staff mainly works 12-hour shifts? Or does the charge nurse work a different length of shift than your staff? Understanding that the charge nurse's schedule can improve your day of operations staffing is essential.

As you learned earlier, charge nurses spend much time on intra-shift staffing. So have your charge nurses come in an hour before the change of the staff nurse shifts. There are several benefits to having charge nurses start earlier than staff shift change. The charge nurses can do the following:

- Hand off important issues among themselves with fewer interruptions.

- Focus on their incoming staff.

- Plan effectively for staffing before the staff arrives.

- Be there throughout the shift to see how well (or not so well) their plan worked.

Another benefit is that the staff understands the expected patient volume for the day.

Some organizations may have the outgoing charge nurse prepare the staffing assignments for the oncoming shift. There are some arguments to support this practice, such as the fact that the off-going charge nurses know the unit's patients better as they have just spent the entire shift with them. The concern is that they may need to learn the oncoming staff's ability, and they are not staying on the shift to see how the staff directly impacted the flow of that shift.

A typical point of confusion is that your charge nurses may take a patient assignment. This now affects your direct and indirect time. How do you consider a working charge nurse's time for budgeting for direct and indirect hours? Most benchmarking organizations place all the hours into the direct care bucket for individuals who work in direct patient care 50% of the time or more. If your organization can split individuals into both direct and indirect buckets, then by all means, do that. If not, follow this calculation to determine the percentage of time your charge nurse or support staff represents direct and indirect care. To define the position(s) as a percentage, divide the required indirect time by the direct time and multiply by 100%:

Indirect time ÷ Direct time =

240 minutes ÷ 480 minutes x 100% =

50%

Understanding your direct and indirect hours and costs is important to support your FTE needs and staffing. Ensure you count every staff member appropriately in the right bucket so your data is as clean as possible.

Maintaining Staff Morale

Scheduling can be a very heated and political topic regardless of where or how long you have worked there. Unfortunately, for those of you who are conflict-averse, this can harm your morale. So, how do you deal with these issues? If you have a shared leadership committee, these are the types of decisions that the committee should help make. Whatever decision it makes, you need to own it. You cannot delegate your responsibility as the manager to the shared leadership team, mainly to have it make a decision you do not want to make.

> **TIP**
>
> *If you make someone happy, you have probably upset someone else. You cannot make everyone happy all the time. Your job as the manager is to be friendly to your staff, not to be friends with your staff.*

You should have a clear process written down in a policy or procedure guide about scheduling components such as tradeoffs, signing up for shifts, holiday rotations, and weekends. In order to maintain morale, you need to have a process that is fair to all staff but consistent with human-resource policies and organizational expectations. Suppose the organization supports the scheduling process by seniority. Those with the most seniority can sign up first for holidays and other preferred days.

In an attempt to retain all staff, many organizations have moved away from rewarding employee seniority. Rewarding seniority recognizes the nurses who have stayed at an organization the longest. However, it is fraught with issues. Is seniority measured from the time of hire, no matter what positions they had first? Does it start when they become RNs? Does it measure only time on that unit? A senior nurse on one unit may be someone other than a senior nurse on another. Treating all staff equally does have its issues, but staff at all levels will feel they are being treated fairly.

Building the Initial Schedule

Say you treat all staff the same. How do you go about creating a fair schedule? Consider these methods for decreasing "scheduling hogs," assessing tradeoffs, and determining vacation days and holidays.

Initial scheduling is complex. With an electronic scheduler where staff log on and choose their scheduled days, you can build many rules to decrease work after staff members enter their desired days. If you are on paper schedules, ensure everyone is aware of the processes and that they stick to them.

Here are two options for structured staff involvement in scheduling:

- Post the open schedule to your full-time staff first, then your part-time staff, and then your per diem staff, allowing for several days in between. This may seem unfair, but remember that full-time employees need more hours than the other two groups. They also have a more significant FTE requirement for your unit.

- Place your staff in two to five equal groups: full-time, part-time, and per diem staff. When you open the schedule, open it first to group 1, followed by groups 2 and 3. Then, for the next open scheduling period, group 2 gets to be first scheduled, followed by group 3, then group 1. Continue to repeat. This way, each group is equal and rotates through everyone, decreasing a scheduling-hog effect.

However you decide to structure staff involvement, you must remain consistent, fair, and vigilant in monitoring staff concerns. All your staff may not like the process, but as long as they know that the rules are the same for everyone and there is no favoritism, they will respect the process.

Maximum Hours and Shifts

Adding to the complexity is whether to limit the number of hours or how many shifts in a row your staff can sign up for. There are night-shift RNs who prefer to schedule themselves on Thursday, Friday, and Saturday of one week and Sunday, Monday, and Tuesday of the following week—working their required shifts full time but working six days in a row. Understandably, night staff want to flip back to days during their off time, giving them that flexibility. However, research shows that deaths from pneumonia were significantly more likely in hospitals where nurses reported schedules with long hours and a lack of time away from work (Aiken et al., 2011). Additionally, certain mortality rates were associated significantly with hours per week and days in a row worked (Aiken et al., 2011).

Consider creating a policy that limits staff from working more than four 12-hour shifts in a row without a 24-hour break before a fifth shift and requires staff to be off for at least 10 hours between shifts. The Occupational Safety and Health Administration (2024) warns against working more than 8-hour shifts due to reduced alertness. The Department of Veterans Affairs Health Care Personnel Enhancement Act of 2004 encourages the Secretary of Veterans Affairs to limit work hours of nurses providing direct patient care in excess of 12 consecutive hours or more than 60 hours in any seven-day period, except in the case of nurses providing emergency care (Department of Veterans Affairs, 2004). While five 8-hour shifts may not be appealing—some staff RNs reported feeling they were always at work (Maust-Martin, 2015)—consider other options, such as four 8-hour shifts or four 10-hour shifts.

This policy will be controversial initially, but no one can argue against patient safety. The policy allows nurses to pick up additional shifts at a neighboring hospital. As the manager, though, you have control over only your unit and an ethical responsibility to keep patients safe. Nurses who decide to pick up extra shifts are making a choice that could jeopardize patient safety and their licenses.

Vacation Days

For vacations, always start with understanding your organization's policy. Make sure you have the following questions answered, or ensure that you answer them in your staffing and scheduling policy—with the input of staff members if they can have input in this matter:

- Is there a set time frame for requesting vacation or paid time off (PTO)? For example, staff must request vacation days or PTO at least six months before being off.

- What is the maximum amount of time anyone can take off at one time?

- Can staff members request vacation time even if they do not have enough hours at the time of the request to cover the days off? What if they need more hours when the vacation comes?

- How many staff can you allow to take vacation at one time?

- Did you figure in your unit's average sick calls, FMLA, and LOAs when determining how many staff can have vacation time at once?

- Will the float pool be able to meet your needs to replace your staff on vacation?

- Do you have the slack in staff to cover the vacation time without outside unit help?

- Does your organization allow vacation time during and around holidays?

Once you have those questions answered and understand your needs and abilities, you can figure out who gets it! Here are two practical methods:

- One method is first come, first served. This method is fair for those who know what they are doing months in advance but less fair to those who have an event turn up at the last minute. You know your staff: the planners and those who live life one day at a time. Before you say that people need to plan better, remember your morale and that some tendencies like these are innate to who they are as people.

- Another method is to open vacation requests whenever you like, but wait to consider all requests until right before the schedule opens. Now, if you complete a schedule one month at a time and post two weeks before, that is an issue for those wanting plane tickets. Consider building a one- to two-month schedule posted two to four weeks before. As you consider those requests, consider what that staff requested for last year and the reason. You will have staff who know their wedding dates a year out. Are you going to deny their requests? Probably not. Some individual judgment is involved, but if staff members understand your reasons for doing what you do, they will consider it fair even though they may not like it.

> **Consider This**
>
> You will still need to smooth the schedule before it is posted. Make sure that staff members meet their FTE requirements, weekend requirements, holidays, and vacation needs. Ensure the staff knows the schedule is only final once it is posted. Too often, staff takes an initial version and fails to check the final version. Also, have a process in place to notify the staff in case a change is made after the official posting of the schedule. Once posted, it is unfair to make a change without letting the staff know.

A close relative of vacation time is personal request days. A personal request day may be considered like a vacation day in your organization, where staff members must take their vacation time to cover the day. A personal request day is used mainly to request a single day off for a physician appointment or other personal reasons. With a personal request day, staff would still be required to work to their FTE in that given work week if not required to use their vacation time. Occasionally, staff may abuse this process, using it to get the days off they want without having to use vacation or sick time, so as the unit manager, you will need to monitor this process for abuse. If done correctly, this process will improve staff members' satisfaction with scheduling, as they can improve their work-life balance without needing to use vacation time for non-vacation-time reasons.

Staff vacation time is very important, and it is a delicate balance for the staff in asking for time off and confirming plans for personal or vacation time. Although this can be an emotional issue, especially if the request is denied, remember that the process needs to remain consistent and fair to all staff.

Holidays

Only a few people like working the holidays, so you will always have someone unhappy about working one. To make it easier, involve staff members in this process to determine how they want to staff holidays. What is your organization's policy on holidays? Start with ensuring that your holiday list includes what your organization considers a major and/or minor holiday. Many organizations state that staff has to work one or two major and minor holidays a year. Also, is there leeway to add additional unit holidays? Do you have a unit where there are many staff with young kids? Maybe everyone wants Halloween or the day after Thanksgiving off. Have your staff members determine whether unit-specific holiday rotation is needed. You can add it on top of their organizational requirement.

An added complexity to holidays is your night staff. What the day staff may consider a holiday may be different from the night staff. Remember that your staff involvement in this will include both day and night staff. Here are two options for staffing night staff around holidays:

- The easiest method is to track who worked which holidays from the prior year and let them take them off this year. However, what do you do if you have staff who transferred from another unit who had to work it last year and are requesting it off? Not an easy call.

- Another way is to divide your staff into groups again—1, 2, and 3 (or as few or as many as you need to cover the days)—and assign holidays in blocks (see Table 8.2). This year, group 1 works holiday group 1, and next year, group 1 works holiday group 2. As staff are hired, you add them to the holiday group in which they are needed; this way, you can let them know upfront what their holiday commitment will be. Based on night staff, you might have Holiday Day groupings and Holiday Night groupings. Remember that your number of groupings is based on the number of staff you have and how many you need to cover each day and night shift.

TABLE 8.2 EXAMPLE HOLIDAY DAY GROUPINGS

Holiday Group 1	Holiday Group 2
Christmas Eve Day (major holiday)	Christmas Day (major holiday)
New Year's Eve Day (major holiday)	New Year's Day (major holiday)
Thanksgiving Day (major holiday)	July 4th (major holiday)
Labor Day (minor holiday)	Memorial Day (minor holiday)
Mother's Day (unit-chosen holiday)	Halloween (unit-chosen holiday)

Again, get staff input on the holiday schedule and rotation. Which nonholidays are important to your staff? Is it the same every year? Remember, a fair and consistent holiday process is just as important as the overall schedule.

Trading Shifts

Tradeoffs should be straightforward; however, there is always the he-said, she-said aspect. Someone thought they made a trade in a shift with another person, and somehow, the other person really did not agree or forgot. Create a process that allows tradeoffs after the schedule is closed and posted. This process should include the following items:

- Create a policy or unit guideline so staff understand that tradeoffs cannot create overtime or shift incentives for someone.

- It is the responsibility of the person wanting to trade a shift to find someone to trade with, to complete the process, and to work the shift if they do not find someone to trade with.

- Create a tradeoff document that states the name of the person wanting to trade, the person who will take the trade, the dates of the trade(s), the specifics of the policy that need to be reinforced (e.g., cannot create overtime), a spot for each person's signature, and a spot for your signature. A trade is only considered approved once all signatures have been obtained. Ensure your staff knows this includes your signature because you need to assess the tradeoff before approval.

- Allow only yourself (or your designee) to change the final schedule. The last thing you want is staff writing all over a posted schedule. If you have an electronic schedule, the same thing—allow only yourself (or your designee) to approve and make the change there as well.

Your staff needs the ability to trade shifts as needed with your oversight. The manager needs to help staff members balance their work and private lives. A policy that clearly outlines the process will ensure a fair and transparent trading process within guidelines that prevent trades that would lead to things such as excessive overtime or taking advantage of incentive pay.

Low Census

Now you have mastered the perfect schedule; you have managed your resources and did not overhire; flu season was not as bad this year (natural variability); and you have fewer patients. However, now you have to deal with the low census. Some staff members hate low census, while others want it daily.

Again, start with your organization's policy on low census and conform to it. However, there might be specifics that you need to manage on your unit. Here are some considerations for managing low census:

- Create a log on the unit that charge nurses manage to keep track of all staff members, what dates they took a low census, and who had a low census last.

- Take turns. You may have people who always want a low census. Pass it around to staff members who like and request that option. Nevertheless, that group still needs to take turns getting it.

- Work with the centralized staffing office or other units before you grant low census. Are the other units covered sufficiently?

- Ensure that you have covered this topic and the process of the low census for your unit, and always incorporate your staff in this topic.

Managing your resources (artificial variability) will help keep your low-census days low so that you do not burden your staff with unnecessary days off. Most people work because they need money and would instead not take their vacation days to cover a low-census day.

Multiple Shift Lengths

Having multiple shift lengths seems like a way to create more chaos in your schedule; however, it can help to fill shifts. Multiple shift lengths can also create confusion for staff and patients, so they must be managed well. Here are some excellent reasons to consider having multiple shift lengths:

- You have older or retired nurses who may not be able to work a 12- or 8-hour shift but can work part of a shift to cover full-shift nurses while they take breaks or lunch.

- You can alternate long and short shifts for older or retired nurses to give them a break between long days for increased rest.

- You can bring in a nurse during the four hours of highest admissions and discharges to improve patient flow.

- You need to fill an open shift day of operations, and you can get two staff to cover one shift.

- You have a great shared leadership committee and involvement. However, the meetings are the same day as the staff's direct-care day. Having a four-hour shift might allow your staff members to attend their committee meeting (and it demonstrates your commitment to shared leadership).

- You have a few nurses who want to job share or split a position—two nurses work the same days, with one working the first half of the shift and the other nurse the second half.

- Short shifts are less conducive to taking a patient assignment but work better when tasks or functions are assigned to this nurse. If a nurse takes an assignment on a short shift, plan to cover those patients once the nurse is done with the short shift instead of making the nurse stay longer.

- Many of these ideas suggest older or retired nurses, but there may be a nurse with daycare issues who can work the same short shifts to give breaks to staff.

Novel Holiday Solution That Did Not Go as Planned

I was a manager of a small ICU in a community hospital where most of my new RNs in the ICU were hired at the same time. As the holidays approached, the hospital's holiday policy and intense political overtones began affecting the newly hired ICU nurses. The hospital's past holiday policies were basic and had worked well for that small community hospital. The policy gave staff members who were employed the longest the days off that they wanted. For that reason, the long-standing hospital policy was not going to work for the ICU. The newly hired ICU nurses were beginning to discuss leaving. Because it was challenging to find RNs who knew basic EKG arrhythmias along with more advanced skills, I wanted to save the newly hired ICU RNs and ensure patient safety during the holidays. We researched holiday staffing policies in surrounding larger communities and city hospitals. Ideas were generated at various nurses' meetings. Some great ideas were discussed during these meetings, voted on, and forwarded to administration. Departmental administrators responded, "Old traditions are hard to break." Finally, I found an article in a nursing management magazine that sounded like a good possibility.

The article presented a possible solution for smaller hospitals' holiday staffing issues that had been highly successful at other community hospitals on the East Coast. The article said to take the 12-hour shifts and break them into 6 hours, and everyone would have to work one 6-hour shift during the holiday. Even though all nurses would work, they would get most of the holiday off. The hospital staff was positive, and the various departments wanted to try the 6-hour shift policy. The administration released a memo stating that the older policy would be replaced if the trial holiday policy of 6-hour shifts was successful over the upcoming holidays.

What happened in the ICU went unbelievably wrong. As the manager, I did not anticipate that politics among the physicians would not mix with the new trial 6-hour shift holiday policy. Without anyone's knowledge, a

> well-loved physician permitted three ICU nurses to change their 6-hour
> shift into 1½- to 3-hour shifts, which was not discovered until the first
> holiday shift. The 6-hour shift holiday policy was successful in all hospital
> departments except the ICU.
>
> –B.S.W.

Multiple shift lengths do not have to add complexity to your schedule. Assess
the needs of your unit and determine how you can best improve the flow or work-
day with a partial-shift employee. Recognize that longer shifts can have a negative
impact on patient and nurse outcomes.

Daily Staffing

We have touched on daily staffing throughout this book and this chapter. If you
have spent the time creating a great schedule, been fair with staffing, managed
your resources, and understood your workforce needs and budget, then you have
done as much as you can up until this point in staffing for quality patient care.

Although you typically own your schedule and staffing process, a centralized staffing office or the house (or administrative) supervisor might own the
day-of-operations staffing. This department or individual is usually responsible
for considering all the happenings in the entire organization to make decisions.
Although you are losing some control over your unit, another unit or department
may be worse off for various reasons. Therefore, getting to know your house
supervisors and those in the centralized staffing department is important. Here
are some important questions to ask them:

- How do they decide to add, float, or low census staff based on patient
  census and volume fluxuations?

- How do they make decisions to place patients?

- Do they know your processes? Your budget and staffing concerns?

- Do they work with your charge nurses? Do your charge nurses work with
  them?

- When do issues need to be escalated up to you?

- Is there an agreement for timely feedback? Telling you about an issue a week later does not enable you to manage it effectively. Conversely, if there is an issue or a staff member who is an issue for them, you need to fix it.

Consider This

Nothing is more irritating than someone saying, "It is not our patient." Staff does it all the time, and managers do it too when protecting their unit. Whether you are in the ED, labor and delivery, ICU, or med-surg, patients who come into the hospital, regardless of where they are or who their nurse is, *are your patients.*

The House Supervisor's Role in Daily Staffing Decisions

Staffing, much like nursing, is both an art and a science. In our health-care world, which is ever-evolving with challenging payer mixes, we must become more creative as we balance patient safety, extraordinary patient care, and RN satisfaction while always keeping budgets at the forefront of our decision-making.

The science side is relatively easy, as a matrix is created based on a budget, and a staffer matches the number of patients with the number of nurses and ancillary staff needed. Sound simple? Not at all, as now the art and experience piece comes in. The decision-maker for staffing, often a house supervisor, must take this snapshot in time and determine how many more patients will be discharged or transferred and how many more will be admitted, along with the acuity of the patients on a nursing unit. Several acuity systems are available on the marketplace, but most require manual data entry and a good deal of interpretation.

> The house supervisor works with the RN managers in the nursing units, the ED, OR, and other procedural areas to determine the anticipated patients for the upcoming shift. They must also work with the nursing staff and the physicians to determine the number of patients we discharge or transfer. Estimate too many, the nursing staff is stretched too thin; estimate too few, a unit is overstaffed, and all eyes are on the decision-maker.
>
> Oh, yes, and do not forget the acuity piece—the house supervisor must be keenly in touch with the skill level of the managers as they evaluate the acuity and needs of the unit. Often, the leader directly influences the flow and stress level of the staff. These are just a few things to consider as the decision-maker balances the art and science of staffing a hospital while always being mindful of the budget.
>
> –Jerri Foster, MSN-L, RN

In the end, remember that everyone has a tough job, and people do not come to work saying they want to do a lousy job. Before thinking that people are out to get you or that they just do not get it, talk to them. People think they make the best decisions they can at the time they make them. If they do not have any feedback, how can they know to improve?

Summary

Here are the key points covered in this chapter:

- A good idea at the wrong time is a bad idea.

- Update your unit's workforce plan every quarter.

- Use shared leadership to engage your staff, improve morale, and get buy-in.

- Change your and your staff's perspective to be aware that all patients are your patients, regardless of where they are currently located.

- Treat all your staff fairly. Create clear documents that outline processes and procedures for staffing.

- Spending the time ahead, managing resources, and planning for your workforce will result in a better end product (schedule).

References

Aiken, L. H., Cimiotti, J., Sloane, D. M., Smith, H. L, Flynn, L., & Neff, D. F. (2011). The effects of nurse staffing and nurse education on patient deaths in hospitals with different nurse work environments. *Medical Care, 49*(12), 1047–1053. https://doi.org/10.1097/MLR.0b013e3182330b6e

Department of Veterans Affairs. (2004). *Health Care Personnel Enhancement Act of 2004: Public law 108–445.* https://www.govinfo.gov/content/pkg/PLAW-108publ445/pdf/PLAW-108publ445.pdf

Dugan Claudio, T. (2004). Questioning workload resources: Measuring your facility's human resources to best evaluate patient care and unit financial needs. *Nursing Management, 35*(10), 30–35.

Labor Management Institute, Inc. (2009). *PSS annual survey of hours report.* https://lminstitute.com/index.php/asoh/

Maust-Martin, D. (2015). Nurse fatigue and shift length: A pilot study. *Nursing Economic$, 33*(2), 81–87.

Occupational Safety and Health Administration. (2024). *Long work hours, extended or irregular shifts, and worker fatigue.* https://www.osha.gov/worker-fatigue

Scherb, C. A., & Weydt, A. P. (2009). Work complexity assessment, nursing interventions classifications, and nursing outcomes classification: Making connections. *Creative Nursing, 15*(1), 16–22. https://doi.org/10.1891/1078-4535.15.1.16

Summers, J. (2016, March 23). *Safe staffing saves lives.* https://silo.tips/download/safe-staffing-saves-lives

Wilson, D. S., Talsma, A., & Martyn, K. (2011). Mindful staffing: A qualitative description of charge nurses' decision-making behaviors. *Western Journal of Nursing Research, 33*(6), 805–824. https://doi.org/10.1177/0193945910396519

PART 3

Staffing Tools and Models

Innovative Care Delivery Models

This chapter examines additional types of unit-level care models, as well as staffing in rural and Critical Access Hospitals (CAHs). As you read this chapter, consider the unique challenges of each model and how they may fit together, whether within the same hospital or across different hospitals within one healthcare system.

Staffing in Rural and Critical Access Hospitals

So what is so innovative about rural hospitals or CAHs? Innovation is not always about the latest or greatest technology or medications. Innovation is also about contributing to ideas and solutions to workplace challenges. With the size of a CAH, it is not unlike the size of a unit on a bigger hospital, but one unit that sees all types of patients.

There is an inherent bias against nurses working in a CAH. There is a misplaced belief that because the hospital is small, rural, or critical access, nurses do not know how to take care of complex and extremely sick patients. This is far from the truth. These nurses work tirelessly to save patients, often to stabilize them with less medication and technology available to them in an attempt to successfully be transferred to a larger hospital with more resources. CAH staff also will maintain a code for hours until a specialty team can arrive via ambulance because a helicopter or fixed-wing team could not reach the facility in extreme weather conditions. CAH staff are an amazing set of care providers when a patient stays alive for eight or more hours solely because of their care. Critical access and rural nursing is a specialty, and it takes innovation in these settings to give the community the care it needs.

CAH is a designation given to eligible rural hospitals. While you may not be employed in a CAH, you may receive patients from a CAH through transfers or referrals or they may be part of your health system. As you read this chapter, consider the unique challenges of staffing in a CAH and rural setting, and how larger, more urban hospitals may play a role in supporting the CAH nursing practice.

Smaller hospitals face distinct challenges when it comes to staffing and scheduling. Fewer staff and resources, as well as out-of-the-way locations, often play essential roles in these challenges. Small-town and rural hospitals are essential to the health and well-being of people far from major metropolitan areas. As of December 2023, there are 1,366 CAHs in the United States, of which 93% operate in rural areas (Definitive Healthcare, 2019). Approximately 20% of the population, or 60 million people, live in rural areas in the US (Harrington et al., 2020).

Additionally, health disparities such as higher incidence, prevalence, morbidity, mortality, and burden of disease exist in rural America, with life expectancy being over three years less than urban areas (Harrington et al., 2020). The population is also older; 19% of rural residents are over the age of 65, compared to 15% in more urban areas (Harrington et al., 2020). Appropriately so, nursing practice in these settings has been described as different from urban and suburban practice settings due to geographic and social isolation; limited access to human, material, and educational support; and a broader scope of practice with increased responsibility for decision-making and increased social connections to and within the community (MacKinnon, 2012).

Due to these unique challenges and more, CAHs rely disproportionately on government payments due to size, assets, financial reserves, and a higher percentage of Medicare and Medicaid patients. To assist with these challenges, Congress created the CAH designation in 1997 through the Balanced Budget Act to stop CAHs from closing. Due to their unique challenges, Medicare does not include CAHs in the hospital Inpatient Prospective Payment System (IPPS) or the hospital Outpatient Prospective Payment System (OPPS). CAHs are paid for most inpatient and outpatient services to patients at 101% of reasonable costs.

In addition to CAHs, there are several types of rural designations per the Centers for Medicare & Medicaid Services (CMS). This list includes Rural Referral Center, Sole Community Hospital, Low Volume Hospital, Medicare Dependent Hospital, Disproportionate Share Hospitals, as well as a Rural Community Hospital Demonstration (RuralHealth Information Hub, 2023).

Table 9.1 highlights the criteria that define some major differences between rural and CAHs.

TABLE 9.1   DIFFERENCES BETWEEN RURAL AND CRITICAL ACCESS HOSPITALS

Rural	Critical Access Hospital
Fewer than 50 beds	May operate up to 25 beds
	Provides 24-hour emergency services seven days a week
	Average length of stay less than 96 hours (excluding swing bed patients)
Distance from another hospital (more than 30 miles)	More than 35 miles from a hospital or another CAH or more than 15 miles in areas with mountainous terrain or only secondary roads

continues

TABLE 9.1   DIFFERENCES BETWEEN RURAL AND CRITICAL ACCESS HOSPITALS   (CONT.)

Rural	Critical Access Hospital
Located outside of a standard metropolitan statistical area	Located beyond an area of 40,000 or more in population
Rural area	May provide swing beds (CAHs serve individuals needing the type of care generally provided at a skilled nursing facility when the hospital beds are not needed for acute care patients)

Source: Centers for Medicare & Medicaid Services (n.d.); Social Security Administration (n.d.)

The financial health of CAHs is one of the key issues that affect quality, specifically process measures and outcomes (Chatterjee et al., 2021). This leads to little incentive to examine RN staffing and workforce shortages and its relationship to patient outcomes in these settings (Chatterjee et al., 2021). There has been little research on nurse staffing over the last decade in rural and critical access facilities.

Previous data had shown poorer outcomes for rural and CAHs in the past few decades. For instance, mortality rates for heart attack, congestive heart failure, or pneumonia have increased at CAHs, while those rates have declined in other acute care hospitals between 1998 and 2008 (Chen et al., 2009). However, recent research focused on emergency visits shows that despite a 50% increase in ED visits in rural and critical access facilities, the mortality rates are no different than urban area facilities (Greenwood-Ericksen et al., 2021). As in all types of hospitals, RN staffing in CAHs and rural hospitals does impact quality; however, it was noted that LPN and nursing assistant per patient day did not have consistent patterns of impact on hospital quality scores (Davidson et al., 2010).

Prior to the pandemic, hospital administrators in rural and CAHs agreed that the RN shortage was a problem; however, most did not believe the shortage negatively impacted patient care (Cramer et al., 2011). Higher RN hours per patient day in rural hospitals have been associated with higher scores on care quality measures such as pneumonia, heart failure, and acute myocardial infarction (Davidson et al., 2010).

Due to many factors, rural areas have fewer nurses and experience a more significant nursing shortage than urban areas. Geographic regions that experience RN shortages (Cramer et al., 2011):

- Decrease their RN staffing levels

- Increase their LPN hours

- Experience a concurrent drop in hospital patient satisfaction

To better understand issues facing CAHs and rural hospitals, the Nurse Staffing Index (Cramer et al., 2011) was created. It captures the contextual environment regarding nurse skill mix, RN preparation, level of patient care, and RN turnover. Utilizing this instrument, it was found that (Cramer et al., 2011):

- RN staffing is highly variable.

- Overall mean RN-to-patient ratio was within the normal range for medical-surgical units.

- Nine out of 10 CAHs reported days when the ratios were exceeded.

Due to high variability, RN-to-patient ratios do not adequately describe RN workloads in CAHs and rural hospitals. RNs in CAHs must constantly plan and adapt their care and skills to an environment with wide fluctuations in average daily census, inpatient volumes, number of special procedure patients, and levels of care. It is important to note that these factors affect RN workload and patient care (Cramer et al., 2011).

Consider This

It is important to understand how your nurses spend their time. Yen et al. (2018) studied where nurses spend their time:

- Nurses spend only 35% of their time in patient rooms.

- Nurses spend 10% on delegable or non-nursing tasks.

- Nurses spend 25% of their time documenting, regardless of electronic charting usage.

Additionally, RN reassignment was a continuous issue in patient care. RN reassignment entails a greater reliance on less-prepared nursing staff in the inpatient unit during the reassignment. This less-prepared nursing staff member may not be directly supervised by the RN while temporarily reassigned (Cramer et al., 2011).

Transition to Practice

In 2018, the National Academy of Health and the American Academy of Nursing offered an essential policy brief, recommending all new graduate nurses be required to participate in a transition to practice (TTP) residency (Goode et al., 2018). Effective mentors—both formal and informal—play a crucial role in orientation and transition to practice for the new graduate nurse (Zhang et al., 2016). New graduate RN turnover, defined as within the first year after graduation from basic education, is higher than that of RNs who have worked more than one year. It has been noted that up to 50% of nurses will change positions or leave the profession within the first one to two years of practice, with turnover costs associated with each nurse at approximately $52,000 (Waltz et al., 2020).

Once new RNs are "on their own" and no longer need a preceptor, an organization is at greater risk of losing those individuals. From this point to the end of the first year, it is more stressful for RNs and can profoundly impact their career. Some new graduate RN units are dedicated for the first 12 weeks of hire, while others start at the end of the first 12 weeks and continue through the end of the first year.

Accredited residency programs have been shown to have lower turnover rates than nonaccredited programs (Trepanier et al., 2023). The American Nurses Credentialing Center accredits such practice transition programs. TTP residency programs are important in decreasing turnover.

Designated Transition Unit

Our new graduate onboarding is designed as a four-week program in the Designated Transition Unit (DTU), with an additional 6 to 10 weeks in the nurse's home unit. During those four weeks on the DTU, the new graduate RN (NGRN) works with a single preceptor. The preceptor and NGRN "share" the patient assignment, which is four patients, with the NGRN expected to fulfill an increasing assignment over time. This means that in week 1, the NGRN has one patient; in week 2, the assignment is two patients, etc., until the NGRN takes a full load of four patients by week 4. The NGRN is then transferred to their "home" unit for the final 6 to 10 weeks of orientation. The NGRN assignment may return to three patients on the home unit for another week or so. The advanced practice nurse who mentors NGRNs follows each NGRN for 12 months.

The emphasis for the four-week DTU experience is not on accomplishing tasks but on developing clinical judgment, communicating effectively with colleagues and physicians, and setting expectations for continuing professional development.

–Carol Hatler, PhD, RN
St. Joseph's Hospital & Medical Center

Here are three more examples of innovative models for preparing new graduates.

Specialty Training Programs Provide Comprehensive Onboarding of New Grads

Summary: New graduate RNs are hired to select specialty patient care units and attend an extended training program to learn practice standards, skills, and expectations for providing care to that patient population.

Details: Specialty nursing units, such as ICU, Women and Infant Services (WIS), and Periop, have extended training programs. These programs are designed to onboard and train both experienced nurses transferring to the specialty and, when appropriate, carefully selected new graduates. Selected new graduates have been screened and selected based on prior experience (perhaps they were nursing assistants or LPNs in that area previously) and a variety of attributes demonstrated through the interview process. Positive experience in the specialty unit with the new grad as a student is often another factor in the selection process. At hire, the new grads attend the standard new graduate orientation program. They then join the scheduled specialty training program alongside experienced RNs transferring into the specialty. (Timing of the specialty program, new grad orientation, and hire date for the new grads are carefully coordinated whenever possible.) The program may run six weeks or up to six months, depending on the specialty. The new grads attend didactic, skills labs, and precept clinical experiences during this time. Clinical experiences are often on the unit where the new grads have been hired but could also involve rotational assignments to provide a richer learning experience.

Outcome: Careful selection of the right new grad for the specialty unit is the first factor in success for the new grad and the unit. Support from clinical educators, preceptors, unit leaders, and unit staff is critical in supporting the new grad's successful transition into practice. Occasionally, despite best efforts, a mismatch is identified. The best outcome in these cases is transferring the new grad to a less-specialized unit that is a better fit.

Facility-Based Nursing Pool

Summary: New grad RNs are hired into the facility staffing pool to allow for mutual identification of the "best fit" unit.

Details: A small number of new grad RNs (three to five) are selected by a facility committee and placed in the staffing pool for a selected specialty area that encompasses several units, such as WIS. The graduates attend the standardized new graduate training program and the specialty unit training program. The new grads are given a rotational assignment to expose them to all units within the specialty service line. They are assigned to a single unit for a specified period to learn the competencies, practice, and patient care standards of that unit. At the end of that time, they rotate to another related unit until they have completed the training and onboarding program.

Outcome: After the program, the new graduates and the specialty/service line leadership have identified the units that would best benefit and be benefited by the new graduates. The new graduates are moved from the staffing pool to core positions in the identified units.

Nurse Externs

Summary: Student nurses in the last year of their nursing program are competitively selected to participate in a paid nurse extern program.

Details: Senior nursing students apply to a limited number of nurse extern positions. These positions allow soon-to-be new graduates to learn more about the areas of nursing in which they would like to begin their practice. Externs are paid and have a maximum number of hours they can work. The work-hour limit is in place to support the externs in completing their nursing program. During the extern program, the student nurses are allowed to perform skills, with some exclusions, that they have learned and have been validated by their nursing program faculty. Competency verification is also obtained when the nursing students begin their extern program. The program heavily relies on preceptor guidance and decision-making regarding the externs' readiness to take on more responsibilities. The extern program provides an excellent opportunity for nursing students not only to enhance technical skills but also to learn how to assimilate as members of the patient care team. Skills such as communication, interdisciplinary collaboration, and time management are honed during the extern experience.

Outcome: The nurse extern program enhances nursing students' education and facilitates postgraduation transition to practice. The program also allows the nursing student, unit staff, and leadership to determine whether the individual would be successful as a new graduate in that unit. On average, more than 90% of externs are hired as new graduates in the units in which they were externs.

Although there is a mix of innovative structures for new graduate units, here are some of the basics to think about in designing a model of care:

- It should be on a closed medical-surgical unit with or without telemetry capabilities.

- Patients admitted to this unit are aware of the unit and the expertise of the staff and new graduates.

- New graduate RNs may come to the unit after their initial 6- to 12-week orientation with their first preceptor.

- New graduate RNs may spend the first 12 weeks only on this particular type of unit.

- A shift assignment typically starts with one patient and gradually increases; nurses do not take a full patient assignment as they would on a regular unit.

- Additional support staff (often nursing assistants) are utilized as needed.

- Preceptors are staffed in addition to the new graduate RNs.

- Preceptors are chosen based on advanced practice degrees and enthusiasm to teach.

New graduate RNs face many challenges in their first year as nurses. Creating a work environment supporting new graduates in their education and orientation will improve patient outcomes and your new-graduate retention rate.

Collaborative Care Nursing Unit

We have all heard at least one patient say, "Why are you asking me this information *again*?" A patient typically poses this question when the physician and nurse have independently asked for the same information and entered it into their medical record sections—not necessarily collaborating to create a joint plan of care with the patient. Then, the admission assessment or plan of care may not be completed until up to 24 hours after admission, often one-third of the way into the patient's complete stay. In response to this issue, one organization created a collaborative care nursing unit to change how inpatient care was delivered to patients. This change in the care delivery model was part of the Institute for Healthcare Improvement's Transforming Care at the Bedside initiative. In this model, an RN, pharmacist, and physician meet with each patient within 90 minutes of admission. Actual benefits of this model include (ThedaCare, 2024):

- Plan of care created so that all staff and the patient and family know and understand

- Decreased cost of care by 30%

- Reduced waste that occurs when the patient and family separately give information to each provider multiple times

- Decreased average length of stay by 20%

- Increased patient and nurse satisfaction

Although there are many benefits to a collaborative care unit, Table 9.2 notes some additional considerations for staffing and budgeting.

TABLE 9.2 BENEFITS AND POTENTIAL ISSUES FOR COLLABORATIVE CARE UNIT

Benefits	Potential Issues
Decreased time spent by multiple nurses in completing plan of care and admission assessment	Staffing with budget but also allowing an RN to meet within 90 minutes of patient admission
Increased time spent by multiple nurses in completing plan of care and admission assessment	Staffing with physician/hospitalist and pharmacy to meet together within 90 minutes of patient admission
Increased and improved delegation of tasks to LPNs and NAPs (increased use of lower-cost care providers)	Potential resources shifted away from other patients in order to maintain the 90-minute goal if staff members are expected to care for patients on other units
Decreased RN turnover	

Variable Acuity Unit

A variable acuity unit (VAU), acuity adaptable unit (AAU), or universal care patient room is a type of unit where a patient can stay in the same hospital bed for ICU, progressive care, and medical care as they step down in acuity, as opposed to changing beds for those different services. In Arizona for instance, the Department of Health refers to it as a multi-organized service unit (MOSU). In other states, it may be called a universal bed, flexible monitoring, or acuity adaptable. There are multiple names for a VAU based on your state licensing regulations. VAU is a type of licensed bed, and regulations in your state may or may not allow this type of bed.

The care comes to the patient as opposed to the patient moving to the care, truly a patient-centered focus. VAU may be used in a smaller hospital, where providing service in separate intensive care, progressive/telemetry, and medical-surgical units may need to be more efficient and effective.

This can be both a unit-specific model of care and an organizational-level model of care. The adaptable acuity model requires additional training of nursing staff who can support the flexing up and down of acuity. Staffing models will need to adjust, as staffing assignments may need to change throughout the day (Cecconi & Bilkovski, 2023). The variable care delivery model by rural and smaller community hospitals allows them to provide care that aligns with available nursing resources.

Research shows this care delivery model decreases nurse floating and cancellations due to low census, with improved patient satisfaction (Paulik Ramson et al., 2013). There is also an opportunity to see a decrease in worked hours per patient day with a corresponding salary reduction due to improvement in appropriate staff utilization (Paulik Ramson et al., 2013).

In a new hospital, *not* a replacement build, this type of unit may offset the costs of maintaining separate units while census builds. A hospital can be built with something other than VAUs to provide this type of service; most private rooms can be fitted with the necessary equipment and supplies to make it appropriate for intensive care services. This bed type may be used in a specialty hospital or department, such as cardiac services.

One Chief Nurse Executive's Experience With an MOSU

Cathy Townsend, MSN-L, RN, was the chief nursing officer when Banner Ironwood Medical Center (BIMC), a new medical center, opened. When the hospital opened, Townsend was intimately involved with developing the MOSU—a 24-bed critical, progressive, and medical-surgical care unit. Staffing for an MOSU is a dynamic process based on acuity; however, ratios do not exceed 1:2 for critical care patients, 1:4 for progressive care patients, and 1:6 for medical-surgical patients. Those numbers are considered for staff, who may have pure ICU patients (low- to moderate-acuity critical care; higher acuity is transferred out) or a mix of ICU and progressive care or medical-surgical patients. Productivity targets, developed with the help of a process engineer, currently range between 9.8 and 11.5 hours per patient day. Over time, the RNs who practice on the unit are trained in all areas of the MOSU, including critical care, progressive care, and medical-surgical care. A few RNs can even float to the newborn nursery and emergency department. Cross-training at this level requires extensive education. Education is through an accumulated process, with the mindset of "What can you learn today?" through observation, bedside tasks, fellow nurses, and visits to more extensive sister facilities.

Lessons learned: When BIMC opened, several ICU-trained nurses were hired for the unit; however, turnover was high for these RNs because it took more work for them to flex to the lower acuity and higher ratio if needed. Today, progressive and medical-surgical nurses are hired and trained for the ICU. To progress to ICU training, the RNs must demonstrate proficiency in medical-surgical and progressive care, typically a year after hire. ICU training occurs at a sister facility for 8 to 12 weeks.

The RNs who work there love the variety. The patients and families are pleased because they love staying in the same room and seeing the same staff. As the hospital grows, the MOSU unit with critical care will be reconsidered. There have been at most five critical care patients on any given shift; however, as that census increases to eight and ten, consideration for opening a separate critical care unit will begin, leaving the MOSU for progressive care and medical-surgical care only.

A list of benefits and potential issues for a VAU are noted in Table 9.3.

TABLE 9.3 BENEFITS AND POTENTIAL ISSUES FOR VAU

Benefits	Potential Issues
Decreased costs because staff time was not needed to transfer patients between units	Difficulty in training RNs at all levels of care
Improved safety by decreasing the number of personnel communicating around care	Need for surveillance and alarm notification
Improved patient and family comfort and decreased unease	Floor/unit layout without space for monitoring
Improved staff satisfaction due to a variety of care and learning experiences	
Decreased loss of patient personal belongings	
Decreased length of stay	

VAUs bring the nurse and resources to the patient. This type of care delivery model would be one to consider for smaller hospitals or service lines that want to streamline care.

Observation Unit

Observation units are not new, but they can be innovative and significantly impact your unit's staffing, whether staffing for the observation unit or staffing your unit if your hospital has an observation unit. Only one-third of US hospitals have observation units (Lam et al., 2021). It is essential to know that there is a large reimbursement difference between patients billed as "inpatients" and those billed as "observation" or "outpatients," even if they are in an inpatient hospital bed. Inpatient and outpatient or observation have legal definitions for billing as set by CMS and in partnership with what the admitting provider orders.

These short-stay patients, defined as those who stay in the hospital less than 24 hours, mixed in with longer-staying patients create a higher churn for your unit, increasing your RNs' workload of admitting and discharging and decreasing your overall unit's length of stay, which may give a false sense of acuity or care needs. When implementing an observation unit, it is important to separate it from inpatient-designated patients. When observation and inpatients are mixed, care delivery will default to one standard of care across all patient types, leading to more expensive care provided, possibly unnecessarily to observation patients. Some research has concluded that hospitals lost money primarily because reimbursement for observation stays did not cover the cost of care (Sheehy et al., 2013).

If you have inpatient and observation patients mixed in your unit, you will increase your staff's workload. Separating these patients will positively impact the staffing and finances of your unit and hospital, as you will be able to manage the care delivery model differently for each of these groups.

Outcomes noted for dedicated observation units include (Lam et al., 2021):

- 17% to 44% decreased likelihood of admission following observation care

- 23% to 38% shorter length-of-stays in the hospital

- $950 million in annual national cost savings

RN staffing for observation units may be a 1:5 ratio, with processes and paperwork or computer work such as assessments streamlined for efficiency to match the requirements and needs of a short-stay patient. Decreasing or eliminating short-stay patients on an inpatient unit does have implications for staffing and patient flow, as noted in Table 9.4.

TABLE 9.4   BENEFITS AND POTENTIAL ISSUES FOR OBSERVATION UNIT

Benefits	Potential Issues
Decreased staff confusion about admitting and discharge paper/computer work needs between observation and inpatient patients	Need dedicated space for unit; may take away from total number of inpatient beds
Improved efficiencies and decreased workload of inpatient RNs, who will have less frequent admissions and discharges	Need to assure oversight by provider for care
Improved efficiencies for observation unit staff, who will be staffed to manage the higher churn of patients, with a decrease in paper/computer work requirements	Need dedicated utilization management and/or case manager to oversee utilization
Evidence-based evaluation and standardized protocols used to stop inpatient admissions	Patients need to understand billing and their financial responsibility may be a percent of charges not a flat fee
Potentially free up more inpatient beds, which will improve patient flow	

Observation units designated for patients in the hospital for less than 24 hours can improve your RN staffing, lessen workload, streamline efficiencies, and save your unit and hospital money.

Emergency Management

Many people think of disasters in terms of their cause. Natural disasters include blizzards, earthquakes, floods, hurricanes, tornadoes, volcanic eruptions, and wildfires. In contrast, unnatural events include major transportation accidents (bus, train, and plane wrecks), environmental disasters (oil and toxic waste spills), and terrorist attacks, such as the September 11, 2001, attacks on the World Trade Center Twin Towers. (How to deal with pandemics, like COVID-19, is discussed in the next section). Overall, the focus on emergency management has increased significantly in the past several decades.

All hospitals should have an emergency management plan. To understand your unit's role and your role as a manager, read your facility's plan first. In addition, many organizations require staff, particularly managers and leaders who might be involved in a disaster, to take emergency management courses offered online by the federal government. The Federal Emergency Management Agency (FEMA) has helpful information on its website (http://www.fema.gov). This site does not provide information on how to staff in a disaster, but it does give you more things to consider.

Although disaster management has little to do with your schedule or daily staffing today, it can be a significant and vital issue if an emergency does happen. Emergencies are not limited to terrorist attacks and natural disasters; they can be brought on by a health epidemic (flu, Ebola, Zika), hospital fire, or some other mass casualty. Are you and your unit ready for the increased volume of patients in an emergency? A literature review highlights a significant gap in nursing research on healthcare disaster ethics, primarily as related to these questions (Johnstone & Turale, 2014):

- What ethical challenges and quandaries do nurses face during a public health emergency or disaster?

- How can nurses best be prepared for ethical responses in extreme conditions?

- Is it possible for nurses to prepare for catastrophic mass casualty events?

- What is considered sufficient ethical preparedness?

- Can we ensure the ethical behavior of nurses in future events?

- How much personal risk and self-sacrifice is reasonable and justified?

During the Ebola crisis, nurse staffing was one of many significant considerations. In events like this, organizations must ensure enough staff is immediately available to provide intensive care unit-level nursing care in full isolation (Matlock et al., 2015). During the 2014 Ebola crisis, it turned out that staffing a unit for one critically ill patient required 16.8 FTEs for one week of 24/7 care, which is approximately four nurses per shift, to ensure safety (Matlock et al., 2015). The National Institutes of Health clinical center used only volunteers to staff the specialty clinical studies unit until the crisis was over.

Consider This

Many nurses are concerned about whether they are legally responsible to respond in a disaster. In some states, nurses are legally bound to respond, so it is essential to talk with your state board of nursing to understand your and your staff's roles in this situation. Whether or not staff are legally bound to help will significantly impact your ability to staff and provide quality patient care, especially since the beginning phases of a disaster can last days to weeks.

Only a little research exists on nursing, nurse staffing, and disaster management, but case studies are available for guidance. Although different types of disasters place different demands on resources, one recommendation from a study found that nurse-to-physician staffing is typically two to one for field hospital and on-scene triage (Yin et al., 2012). Ratios for your unit may vary based on which patients you will receive from a disaster or your role in helping other units. These are considerations related to staffing during a disaster:

- Ensure you have updated contact information (phone numbers and street addresses) for all your staff. Know which staff members communicate via text, as well as other chat messaging systems such as Teams. When land and cell lines become overrun with calls, texting may be the only way to contact your staff outside of work.

- Develop a list of nurses with four-wheel drive vehicles (in adverse weather).

- Develop a pick-up list, in case of adverse weather, that identifies which nurses can pick up other nurses to drive to and from work.

- Understand which nurses have family commitments that may come first during a disaster. Who will need to secure care for a child, elder, or pet before they can come in to help?

- Know whether staff members can come in if you can assist them with their family and personal responsibilities.

- List people who do not have other responsibilities that would prevent them from coming in.

- Determine whether there is space for staff members to sleep at the hospital or in the unit in case they cannot leave.

- Ensure that food and water are available for staff who stay during an emergency.

- Know where disaster supplies (extra protective gear, etc.) are kept at the hospital.

- Determine whether your facility has tents if triage outside the facility is necessary.

No one knows when a disaster will strike, and no area is safe from a disaster. The best plan is to be prepared for anything. Understand your hospital's emergency plan and how your unit will be able to respond in partnership with the plan.

Pandemic Response

Most of us had never experienced a pandemic, particularly as healthcare providers, until COVID-19. The one thing we know is that this will not be the last time we experience a pandemic. In fact, the World Health Organization (WHO) states that the end of COVID-19 as a global health emergency is not the end of COVID-19 as a global health threat (UN News, 2023), further noting that "when the next pandemic comes knocking—and it will—we must be ready to answer decisively, collectively, and equitably" (UN News, 2023, para. 2). WHO launched the PRET initiative and a Global Call to Action to strengthen preparedness by (WHO, 2023):

- Updating national pandemic plans
- Increasing connectivity among stakeholders
- Ensuring dedicated investments in pandemic preparedness

With this, the most important item to take away is that we all spend time reflecting globally, nationally, and locally within our organization. Evaluate how your organization handled (and is still handing) COVID-19: what worked and what you might need to do again. Refine those things that were beneficial and incorporate them into your emergency and pandemic response policies. Do not let those lessons be forgotten.

With COVID-19, approximately 5% of infected patients needed critical care, and 30% of those required admission in an intensive care unit (Schwerdtle et al., 2020). This created more need than capacity for admissions to acute care. Many organizations needed to create space, thus capacity, to provide care in areas that do not normally provide care. In organizations, this may have been overflow units or surgical areas, and it is vitally important to have those areas maintain readiness for events like this. These areas may be staffed with float staff, and they may not have supplies stocked and ready to go. In addition to treating these areas as overflow, treat them as an emergency or pandemic response unit. Consider what staff may float to this unit, what skill sets and competencies may be required, and work to always be prepared to use this area. It could also be incorporated as the site for emergency response drills within the facility.

Another lesson from the pandemic and benefit to having roster management is that reports can be run quickly to vital data. Many hospitals needed more ICU nurses or nurses who could manage ventilators. Some hospitals could run a report to be able to see all their employed staff that had transferred out of the ICU in the prior year to understand who has worked ICU recently enough that they could come back to the ICU and take a regular patient assignment immediately. Reports could also be run to determine whether nurses with a past history of ICU experience could quickly be partnered with a current, experienced ICU nurse. Additionally, hospitals created functional nurse teams that covered the entire hospital and completed tasks like IV starts.

Like any prolonged emergency, nurses have been faced with higher levels of burnout and turnover than ever before during and after COVID-19. It is important to note that these issues did not occur because of COVID-19, but over several decades of poor staffing, scheduling, and workforce shortages that went mostly unaddressed. This is why it is so important to improve your staffing and scheduling now. As it has been noted, another pandemic will occur.

Summary

- Rural and Critical Access Hospitals have distinctive characteristics and are vital to the healthcare delivery system.

- Skilled management and willingness to change are necessary to implement innovative practices successfully.

- Always involve your staff.

- New ways of providing care still need to be developed!

- Discuss and understand disaster management.

- Reflect on pandemic response and incorporate lessons learned into your policies.

References

Cecconi, M., & Bilkovski, R. (2023). *Adaptable acuity care models: A path forward for future global health system challenges.* GE HealthCare. https://clinicalview.gehealthcare.com/sites/default/files/MS%20Clinical%20View%20white%20paper%20Adaptable%20Acuity.pdf

Centers for Medicare & Medicaid Services. (n.d.). *Critical Access Hospitals.* cms.gov/medicare/health-safety-standards/certification-compliance/critical-access-hospitals

Chatterjee, P., Werner, R. M., & Joynt Maddox, K. E. (2021). Medicaid expansion alone not associated with improved finances, staffing, or quality at Critical Access Hospitals. *Health Affairs, 40*(12), 1846–1855. https://doi.org/10.1377/hlthaff.2021.00643

Chen, C., McNeese-Smith, D., Cowan, M., Upenieks, V., & Afifi, A. (2009). Evaluation of a nurse practitioner–led care management model in reducing inpatient drug utilization and costs. *Nursing Economic$, 27*(3), 160–168.

Cramer, M. E., Jones, K. J., & Hertzog, M. (2011). Nurse staffing in Critical Access Hospitals: Structural factors linked to quality care. *Journal of Nursing Care Quality, 26*(4), 335–343. https://doi.org/10.1097/NCQ.0b013e318210d30a

Davidson, G., Belk, K., & Moscovice, I. (2010). *Nurse staffing and rural hospital performance improvement.* Upper Midwest Rural Health Research Center. http://rhrc.umn.edu/wp-content/files_mf/davidsonnursestaffing.pdf

Definitive Healthcare. (2019). *Rural America's health crisis: Critical-access & safety net hospitals.* https://www.definitivehc.com/blog/critical-access-safety-net

Goode, C. J., Glassman, K. S., Ponte, P. R., Krugman, M., & Peterman, T. (2018). Requiring a nurse residency for newly licensed registered nurses. *Nursing Outlook, 66*(3), 329–332. https://doi.org/10.1016/j.outlook.2018.04.004

Greenwood-Ericksen, M., Kamdar, N., Lin, P., George, N., Myaskovsky, L., Crandall, C., Mohr, N. M., & Kocher, K. E. (2021). Association of rural and Critical Access Hospital status with patient outcomes after emergency department visits among Medicare beneficiaries. *JAMA Network Open, 4*(11), e2134980. https://doi.org/10.1001/jamanetworkopen.2021.34980

Harrington, R. A., Califf, R. M., Balamurugan, A., Brown, N., Benjamin, R. M., Braund, W. E., Hipp, J., Konig, M., Sanchez, E., & Joynt Maddox, K. E. (2020). Call to action: Rural health: A presidential advisory from the American Heart Association and American Stroke Association. *Circulation, 141*(10), e615–e644.

Johnstone, M. J., & Turale, S. (2014). Nurses' experiences of ethical preparedness for public emergencies and healthcare disasters: A systematic review of qualitative evidence. *Nursing and Health Sciences, 16*, 67–77. https://doi.org/10.1111/nhs.12130

Lam, C. (2021, Feb. 3). Financial impacts of ED observation units: Literature and strategies review. *EMResident.* https://www.emra.org/emresident/article/lit-review-observation-units

MacKinnon, K. (2012). We cannot staff for 'what ifs': The social organization of rural nurses' safeguarding work. *Nursing Inquiry, 19*(3), 259–269. https://doi.org/10.1111/j.1440-1800.2011.00574.x

Matlock, A. M., Gutierrez, D., Wallen, G., & Hastings, C. (2015). Providing nursing care to Ebola patients on the national stage: The National Institutes of Health experience. *Nursing Outlook, 63*(1), 21–24. https://doi.org/10.1016/j.outlook.2014.11.015

Paulik Ramson, K., Dudjak, L., August-Brady, M., Stoltzfus, J., & Thomas, P. (2013). Implementing an acuity-adaptable care model in a rural hospital setting. *The Journal of Nursing Administration, 43*(9), 455–460. https://doi.org/10.1097/NNA.0b013e3182a23b9b

RuralHealth Information Hub. (2023). *Rural hospitals.* https://www.ruralhealthinfo.org/topics/hospitals

Schwerdtle, P. N., Connell, C. J., Lee, S., Plummer, V., Russo, P. L., Endacott, R., & Kuhn, L. (2020). Nurse expertise: A critical resource in the COVID-19 pandemic response. *Annals of Global Health, 86*(1). https://doi.org/10.5334/aogh.2898

Sheehy, A. M., Graf, B., Gangireddy, S., Hoffman, R., Ehlenbach, M., Heidke, C., Fields, S., Liegel, B., & Jacobs, E. A. (2013). Hospitalized but not admitted: Characteristics of patients with "observation status" at an academic medical center. *JAMA Internal Medicine, 173*(21), 1991–1998. https://doi.org/10.1001/jamainternmed.2013.8185

Social Security Administration. (n.d.). *Payment to hospitals for inpatient hospital services.* ssa.gov/OP_Home/ssact/title18/1886.htm

ThedaCare. (2024). *Collaborative care: Case study by the Center for Healthcare Value.* https://createvalue.org/collaborative-care/

Trepanier, S., Ogilvie, L., & Yoder-Wise, P. S. (2023). The impact of accreditation on nursing transition into practice residency programs. *Nurse Leader, 21*(3), 349–354. https://doi.org/10.1016/j.mnl.2023.01.004

UN News. (2023, May 22). *World must be ready to respond to next pandemic: WHO chief.* https://news.un.org/en/story/2023/05/1136912

Waltz, L. A., Muñoz, L., Weber Johnson, H., & Rodriguez, T. (2020). Exploring job satisfaction and workplace engagement in millennial nurses. *Journal of Nursing Management, 28*(3), 673–681. https://doi.org/10.1111/jonm.12981

World Health Organization. (2023, July 14). *Welcoming a new era for respiratory pathogen pandemic preparedness in the Western Balkans and the Republic of Moldova.* https://www.who.int/news/item/14-07-2023-welcoming-a-new-era-for-respiratory-pathogen-pandemic-preparedness-in-the-western-balkans-and-the-republic-of-moldova

Yen, P. Y., Kellye, M., Lopetegui, M., Saha, A., Loversidge, J., Chipps, E. M., Gallagher-Ford, L., & Buck, J. (2018). Nurses' time allocation and multitasking of nursing activities: A time motion study. *AMIA Annual Symposium Proceedings, 2018*, 1137.

Yin, H., He, H., Arbon, P., Zhu, J., Tan, J., & Zhang, L. (2012). Optimal qualifications, staffing, and scope of practice for first responder nurses in disaster. *Journal of Clinical Nursing, 21*(1–2), 264–271. https://doi.org/10.1111/j.1365-2702.2011.03790.x

Zhang, Y., Qian, Y., Wu, J., Wen, F., & Zhang, Y. (2016). The effectiveness and implementation of mentoring program for new graduate nurses: A systematic review. *Nurse Education Today, 37*, 136–144. https://doi.org/10.1016/j.nedt.2015.11.027

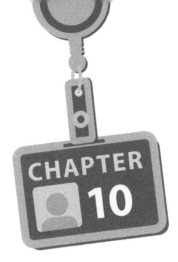

CHAPTER 10

Outside the Hospital Walls

The Patient Protection and Affordable Care Act (ACA) of 2010 had significant implications for the delivery of care, including changing pay structures, so that organizations, such as Accountable Care Organizations (ACOs), are responsible for providing care to patients across the continuum—placing a renewed focus on care delivery in settings outside hospital walls.

Because the US healthcare system has been illness-focused for much of its history, with most patient care occurring within a hospital setting, more research is needed on staffing in non-acute care settings. In the years since the ACA went into effect, we have seen a new emphasis on research that focuses on gaps in understanding the provision of quality patient care—and outcomes—in nonhospital settings. In this chapter, we look at what we know about staffing and outcomes in several nonhospital settings. We need additional research to understand how nurse staffing influences care, workload, and care coordination activities and how these factors may impact patient outcomes in the community.

Outpatient Considerations for Staffing and Care Delivery Models

Predictions agree that as healthcare evolves, nursing work will transition from acute care to non-acute care roles. Eventually, more nurses will practice in the community than in critical care.

Nurses have taken on increased accountability and responsibility in transitional care and care coordination. This includes not only having enhanced responsibility and accountability in traditional settings, such as patients' homes and community-based clinics, but increasingly having roles that enable them to move across healthcare settings, such as from hospitals to patients' homes (Fraher et al., 2015).

Knowing that nurses are a vital part of the healthcare delivery system, we need to consider how their roles and the role of the nurse manager may change to meet the demand for increased outpatient services and decreased inpatient services. There needs to be more research to guide nurse staffing decisions outside of the hospital setting, so nurses and nurse managers must ask guiding questions to get to their local answers. Considerations when planning for future changes with nursing staff include (Mensik, 2007):

- What is an appropriate restructuring of resources in healthcare reform or as an ACO?

- What will future revenue be once healthcare reform is fully implemented?

- How will patient volume for inpatient vs. outpatient service change?

- How will organizations manage the transition from inpatient services to community-based services?

- How will organizations purchase or partner with physician practices, outpatient services, and insurance companies?

This uncertainty has created leadership opportunities for all nurses to participate in conversations that will drive the future of nursing in their organizations.

Ambulatory and Urgent Care

Ambulatory care, or clinic-based care, focuses on providing care to outpatients who do not require urgent or emergency care. Clinics are interprofessional in nature, consisting of providers, medical assistants, and LPNs and/or RNs. In some cases, the role of the clinic-based RN is seen as replaceable with a medical assistant. Unfortunately, not enough research exists yet to understand outcomes from clinics based on role staffing. However, RNs are increasingly taking on the role of care coordinator in many settings (Kim & Marek, 2016). As the complexity of ambulatory and primary care evolves, efforts must be directed towards enabling nurses to focus on their substantial role in care coordination (Karam et al., 2021). This includes finding primary care employment models that would facilitate multidisciplinary teamwork and the delivery of integrated care and guarantee the delivery of intensive yet efficient coordinated care (Karam et al., 2021).

As mentioned in Chapter 1, when determining staffing levels, nurses are given time to complete technical tasks such as IV, medication pass, wound care, and assessments. Unfortunately, little time is allotted for care coordination activities in any setting. This contributes to the nurse managers' lack of understanding about appropriate RN resources needed to obtain the best outcomes in the care coordination role.

Comprehensive Care Coordination: The Many Components

- Medication coordination
- Medical/dental care coordination
- Physical signs and symptoms monitoring
- Durable medical equipment management
- Monitoring of laboratory findings

- Self-management education
- Facilitating communication among healthcare providers, family, and the patient (Kim & Marek, 2016)

Another less understood issue, due in part to a need for more research, is the impact of the outpatient work environment on nurse and patient outcomes. Most research has been done in the acute care setting; however, the concepts of a supportive healthcare environment can be transferred into this setting. It is well documented that a work environment that allows nurses to provide quality care results in better patient outcomes. Outpatient managers will need to advance the outpatient setting work environment forward through the establishment of a supportive physical and interpersonal healthcare environment to develop high-performing interprofessional teams and implement electronic documentation systems to track performance so that patients have more opportunities to receive safe, high-quality, evidence-based care (Haas et al., 2016).

Urgent care is a category of walk-in clinic that treats injuries and illnesses that require immediate care but are not severe enough to require an emergency department (ED) visit. Some organizations have a fast-track section for patients needing urgent care in their EDs. Urgent care facilities not attached to an ED are interprofessional and may or may not have nursing staff. Residents may use urgent care instead of a primary care provider in some communities.

Since there are many models of care for urgent care settings, more data is needed on the effect of nurse staffing on patient outcomes. This is especially true as more healthcare systems purchase or open their own urgent care clinics. Consider how these nurses may interact with primary care clinics, EDs, and hospitals. A systematic review noted that across all developed countries, including the US, urgent care was more frequently used by those over the age of 80 who were more acutely unwell and lacked social support for decision-making behaviors, help with insurance, access to primary care, and geographic differences (Turner et al., 2015). This patient population requires nurse care coordination and supports the need for nurses to be staffed in urgent care clinics.

With care delivery models in ambulatory care evolving more into team-based care, research should focus on the staffing and workload of the entire team while noting the RN's role in good patient outcomes (Anderson et al., 2014). It is essential for nursing to clarify its role as a care coordinator on the team as it evolves. Additionally, we must ensure that electronic health records have robust documentation tools and capture nursing-sensitive outcomes.

Long-Term Acute Care

Long-term acute care hospitals (LTACs) provide complex inpatient services for patients in the recovery phase of severe acute illness. Defined by the Centers for Medicare & Medicaid Services (CMS) as acute care hospitals with average lengths of stay exceeding 25 days, LTACs are one of the fastest-growing care delivery settings in the US (Kahn et al., 2013). While this setting provides care for chronic critical illness, more is needed to know how outcomes might change with less intense nurse and physician staffing (Kahn et al., 2013). The researchers further noted that more intense acute care *early* in the form of LTAC admissions prevented post-acute care use later in admitting patients with chronic critical illness to skilled nursing facilities (SNFs; Kahn et al., 2013). Further cost-effectiveness analysis of nursing services on outcomes is hampered due to nursing services being subsumed in the daily bed charge (Kahn et al., 2013).

Skilled Nursing Facilities/Long-Term Care

Approximately 1.5 million elderly and disabled Americans reside in nursing homes. These residents account for over 25% of documented deaths from COVID-19 (Grabowski & Mor, 2020). In September 2023, the Biden administration with the Department of Health and Human Services, through CMS, proposed a minimum nursing staff standard for nursing facilities participating in Medicare and Medicaid. This is the first of its kind, regulating minimum staffing standards as opposed to legislating them. As of April 2024, the rule was finalized with minimum nurse staffing standards.

Fiscal constraints and the nursing shortage have created lower RN-to-resident ratios and higher RN workloads (Choi et al., 2012) as Medicaid is the dominant payer in long-term care (Gandhi et al., 2021). Unresolved issues have led to average RN turnover rates at 140% in these facilities (Gandhi et al., 2021). Nursing home characteristics, including staffing levels, have been shown to lead to turnover and lower nursing staff job satisfaction (Choi et al., 2012). Additionally, nursing homes in areas with lower per capita income, for-profit status, and higher Medicaid status had higher staff turnover rates (Gandhi et al., 2021).

Despite a large data set of nursing-care quality indicators that have been collected on each resident for decades, there are few studies on the impact of staffing and quality—all during a time in which administrators have long struggled to attract and retain RNs and LPNs, and turnover in long-term care is a widespread issue even more so after the COVID-19 global health emergency. As noted by McGilton and colleagues (2014), most of the retention and work environment research has been done in acute care, and the long-term care environment is markedly different. However, some research in this area does support connections between turnover and outcomes. In one study, researchers noted that turnover was positively associated with the probability of an infection control citation (Loomer et al., 2022).

Efforts to support continuity of care models, such as modular nursing or team nursing, may enhance the quality of care by decreasing turnover (McGilton et al., 2014). However, the impact of these care delivery models on outcomes needs to be studied (McGilton et al., 2014). A study found that facilities where the director of nursing practiced complexity leadership—using good work environment attributes such as including more staff input and shared decision-making—had lower rates of survey deficiencies (McKinney et al., 2016). Additionally, administrators looking to improve RN job satisfaction should implement a self-governance model to allow RNs to develop their own work schedules, among other items (Choi et al., 2012).

One innovative practice in many states is using a medication aide to pass medication. *Medication aides* are certified nursing assistants with additional education based on state requirements that allow them to administer certain medications under the delegation of a licensed nurse. The goal is to free up time for the licensed nurse to tend to the patient's other skilled needs. More than studying staffing levels alone is required in nursing homes; research should also include the composition of staff (Castle & Anderson, 2011). Approximately one-quarter of nursing homes receive deficiency citations due to medication errors or administration (Castle & Engberg, 2007). Research has shown that medication aides did not significantly reduce RN or LPN usage and did decrease the probability that a facility received deficiency citations (Walsh et al., 2014). This is due to laws related to medication aides. Medication aides are allowed in 38 states to administer medication through the supervision of a nurse.

>
> **NOTE**
>
> *Multiple states allow medication aides in nursing homes. Because there is no consistent regulatory body from state to state, start with your state board of nursing for more information. It will point you in the right direction.*

More research in nursing homes and long-term care settings has been occurring. Because this area is quite different from other settings regarding licensed and unlicensed staff, it is necessary to avoid assuming similarities in the work environment and patient outcomes. More research, as suggested, is needed to fully understand the impact of staffing, staffing mix, and outcomes in this setting.

Home Health and Hospice

The terms "home health" and "home care" are often used interchangeably, but they are distinctly different services. Here, we will focus on home health research. *Home health* provides a variety of primarily skilled services (RN, PT, OT, ST, MSW) with nursing assistants and requires the expertise of a licensed professional to oversee the care provided. Medicare and private insurance also cover it. *Home care* is primarily custodial care provided by non-licensed/nonmedical caregivers and is not covered by Medicare or private insurance. The US has approximately 11,400 home health agencies (Centers for Disease Control and Prevention, 2020).

There is more research in home health settings on the work environment, workload, and staffing. The work environment has been measured by adapting acute care–focused survey instruments, including the Essentials of Magnetism (Mensik, 2007), and found that what acute care nurses had perceived as organizational measures of a quality work environment were the same attributes that home health nurses perceived to be good measures. Using the Perceived Nursing Work Environment Scale, researchers have noted that home health organizations can improve nurse retention by improving the work environment and ensuring manageable workloads to facilitate improved work-life balance (Tourangeau et al., 2015).

Like all other settings, an improved work environment in home health agencies improves patient outcomes and reduces hospitalization. Increased productivity requirements adding to nurse workload and caseload, combined with other cost-saving factors, may increase turnover and lead to lower quality. Again, adequate staffing and resources are necessary to provide safe and timely patient care (Jarrin et al., 2014). Research is needed to develop and refine methods for measuring home health nurses' workload and further understand the relationship between workload and patient outcomes (Jarrin et al., 2014).

While hospice is vastly different from home health, many similarities exist in workload, caseload, and work environment. *Hospice* is care given at home to provide comfort for the terminally ill. Less research on the work environment in this setting is available, especially regarding patient outcomes, because hospice nursing care is about easing the patient and their discomfort during the dying process. This provides challenges for quantitative studies related to staffing needs. One study found that for-profits were likelier to have fewer RN full-time equivalents than nonprofit hospice organizations (Cherlin et al., 2010). How this relates to patient outcomes is unknown. Other researchers have noted a need for more available information concerning a hospice's capital, labor, staff visits, and outcomes (Cozad et al., 2016). One study did suggest that hospices create float pools that provide flexibility in weathering workload variability (Cozad et al., 2016).

Home health and hospice agencies will continue to proliferate over the next decade due to the ACA's focus on community-based care and a shift from the traditional acute care delivery model. While some research has studied the home health setting, much more information is needed. As care transitions from acute care to preventive and community services, understanding the components of safe staffing is necessary to obtain good-quality patient care in all settings.

Next Steps

More research is needed in all these settings. Just as in acute care, the nursing work environment in non-acute settings plays a significant role in staffing and patient outcomes. Understanding the impact of RNs in each of these settings will require data on the work environment and workload measures for nursing and other disciplines.

Future ideas for research in these areas include obtaining basic data available for the inpatient acute care setting but still needed in the primary and community settings. Questions include:

1. What is the best ratio of RNs to providers to patients to coordinate appropriate care in a clinic?

2. What is the appropriate number of RN hours per resident needed in an SNF to obtain excellent quality resident outcomes based on Minimum Data Set information?

3. What other staff are needed to supplement RNs' time in long-term care facilities?

4. What is the appropriate caseload for RNs in home health that leads to excellent quality outcomes as evidenced by measures collected on the Outcome and Assessment Information Set (i.e., independence in taking medications, wounds healed, lack of UTIs from catheters, and so on)?

5. What is the appropriate caseload for RNs in hospice that leads to excellent quality outcomes as evidenced by measures on the hospice data set (i.e., pain management, constipation, and so on)?

6. How many visits are appropriate daily for a home health or hospice nurse?

However, we should start making changes before this research is completed. An excellent work environment, where perceived staffing and resource adequacy are high, is a start. One place to start is with the American Nurses Credentialing Center's (ANCC) Pathway to Excellence and Magnet® Recognition programs that help organizations move toward creating a good work environment. Both programs are available to any healthcare setting that employs nurses, not just acute care. Free and low-cost tools can be found on the ANCC website at www.nursingworld.org/organizational-programs.

Summary

- Some research in non-acute care settings points to better patient care with higher RN staffing.

- More research is still needed to understand the work environment in community healthcare settings.

- Resources are available for organizations to act on now instead of waiting for research to be published.

References

Anderson, R., Ellerbe, S., Haas, S., Kerfoot, K., Kirby, K., & Nickitas, D. (2014). In J. Mensik (Ed.), *Excellence and evidence in staffing: A data-driven model for excellence in staffing* (2nd ed.). *Nursing Economic$, 32*(3, Suppl.), 1–36.

Castle, N. G., & Anderson, R. A. (2011). Caregiver staffing in nursing homes and their influence on quality of care: Using dynamic panel estimation methods. *Medical Care, 49*(6), 545–552. https://doi.org/10.1097/MLR.0b013e31820fbca9

Castle, N. G., & Engberg, J. (2008). Further examination of the influence of caregiver staffing levels on nursing home quality. *The Gerontologist, 48*(4), 464–476. https://doi.org/10.1093/geront/48.4.464

Centers for Disease Control and Prevention. (2020). *Data from the 2020 National Post-Acute and Long-Term Care Study.* https://www.cdc.gov/nchs/npals/webtables/overview.htm

Cherlin, E. J.., Carlson, M. D. A., Herrin, J., Schulman-Green, D., Barry, C. L., McCorkle, R., Johnson-Hurzeler, R., & Bradley, E. H. (2010). Interdisciplinary staffing patterns: Do for-profit and nonprofit hospices differ? *Journal of Palliative Medicine, 13*(4), 389–394. https://doi.org/10.1089/jpm.2009.0306

Choi, J., Flynn, L., & Aiken, L. H. (2012) Nursing practice environment and registered nurse job satisfaction in nursing homes. *The Gerontologist, 52*(4), 484–492. https://doi.org/10.1093/geront/gnr101

Cozad, M. J., Lindley, L. C., & Mixer, S. J. (2016). Staff efficiency trends among pediatric hospices, 2002–2011. *Nursing Economic$, 34*(2), 82–89.

Fraher, E., Spetz, J., & Naylor, M. (2015). *Nursing in a transformed health care system: New roles, new rules.* INQRI research brief. https://collections.nlm.nih.gov/catalog/nlm:nlmuid-101679491-pdf

Gandhi, A., Yu, H., & Grabowski, D. C. (2021). High nursing staff turnover in nursing homes offers important quality information: Study examines high turnover of nursing staff at US nursing homes. *Health Affairs, 40*(3), 384–391. https://doi.org/10.1377/hlthaff.2020.00957

Grabowski, D. C., & Mor, V. (2020). Nursing home care in crisis in the wake of COVID-19. *JAMA, 324*(1), 23–24. https://doi.org/10.1001/jama.2020.8524

Haas, S. A., Vlasses, F., & Havey, J. (2016). Population health management and quality outcomes in ambulatory care settings. *Nursing Economic$, 34*(3), 126–134

Jarrin, O., Flynn, L., Lake, E. T., & Aiken, L. H. (2014). Home health agency work environments and hospitalizations. *Medical Care, 52*(10), 877–883. https://doi.org/10.1097/MLR.0000000000000188

Kahn, J. M., Werner, R. M., David, G., Ten Have, T. R., Benson, N. M., & Asch, D. A. (2013). Effectiveness of long-term acute care hospitalizations in elderly patients with chronic critical illness. *Medical Care, 51*(1), 4–10. https://doi.org/10.1097/MLR.0b013e31826528a7

Karam, M., Chouinard, M. C., Poitras, M. E., Couturier, Y., Vedel, I., Grgurevic, N., & Hudon, C. (2021). Nursing care coordination for patients with complex needs in primary healthcare: A scoping review. *International Journal of Integrated Care, 21*(1). https://doi.org/10.5334/ijic.5518

Kim, T. Y., & Marek, K. D. (2016). Profiling patient characteristics associated with the intensity of nurse care coordination. *Western Journal of Nursing Research.* https://doi.org/10.1177/0193945916661493

Loomer, L., Grabowski, D. C., Yu, H., & Gandhi, A. (2022). Association between nursing home staff turnover and infection control citations. *Health Services Research, 57*(2), 322–332. https://doi.org/10.1177/0193945916661493

McGilton, K. S., Boscart, V. M., Brown, M., & Bowers, B. (2014). Making tradeoffs between the reasons to leave and reasons to stay employed in long-term care homes: Perspectives of licensed nursing staff. *International Journal of Nursing Studies, 51*(6), 917–926. https://doi.org/10.1016/j.ijnurstu.2013.10.015

McKinney, S. H., Corazzini, K., Anderson, R. A., Sloane, R., & Castle, N. G. (2016). Nursing home director of nursing leadership style and director of nursing sensitive survey deficiencies. *Health Care Management Review, 41*(3), 224–232. https://doi.org/10.1097/HMR.0000000000000072

Mensik, J. S. (2007). The essentials of magnetism for home health. *The Journal of Nursing Administration, 37*(5), 230–234. https://doi.org/10.1097/01.NNA.0000269742.40137.a6

Tourangeau, A. E., Patterson, E., Saari, M., Thomson, H., & Cranley, L. (2015). Work related factors influencing home care nurse intent to remain employed. *Health Care Management Review,* 1–11. https://doi.org/10.1097/HMR.0000000000000093

Turner, J., Coster, J., Chambers, D., Cantrell, A., Phung, V.-H., Knowles, E., Bradbury, D., & Goyder, E. (2015). What evidence is there on effectiveness of different models of delivering urgent care? A rapid review. *Health Services and Delivery of Research, 3*(43), 1–160. https://doi.org/10.3310/hsdr03430

Walsh, J. E., Lane, S. J., & Troyer, J. L. (2014). Impact of medication aide use on skilled nursing facility quality. *The Gerontologist, 54*(6), 976–988. https://doi.org/10.1093/geront/gnt085

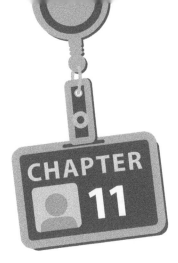

CHAPTER
11

Examples of Staffing Plans, Policies, and Committees

As you have read more about staffing, you have learned how complex and dynamic it is. Having policies and procedures that clearly outline how staffing and scheduling are done is critical so there is a base level of agreement and understanding across the hospital. Some variations may exist for units (based on services provided) as to whether nurses are on call for weekends or work every other, but for the most part, having a standardized approach will treat all staff and managers fairly in the long run.

This chapter provides examples of documents we have discussed in prior chapters. Some examples may not work for you right out of the book; you may have to tweak them to meet your unit's needs. Feel free to take something from one tool and mix it with another. Try different things to see what will work for your situation.

The Importance of Effective Staffing and Staff Input

Healthcare systems face challenges daily around effectively staffing the nursing unit/area to proactively meet the needs of patients while also reducing costs and improving quality. The manager must also consider the model of care needed and evaluate if and how the model supports the structure and function of the dynamics. Integrating evidence-based practice into the hiring process impacts patient care at the highest level. Hiring BSN-prepared RNs does not add to the bottom line, and the patient receives the most prepared caregiver at entry level, thus transcending the care into efficient cost and improved quality.

Another factor that effectively helps nurses on the medical oncology floor is engaging staff in daily decision-making. Currently, staff members use an evidence-based acuity tool to determine care assignments. The acuity tool researched and implemented by our shared governance group at the unit level helps identify patient needs so the charge nurse can match the appropriate assignment with the nurse's experience. Because the tool helps distribute the workload evenly, staff members are more content and less likely to argue about assignments that are too heavy. The onus is then on the charge nurse to use the tool effectively. Happy nurses translate a healthy work environment into higher patient satisfaction as well.

–Donald D. Day, DNP, MSN, RN

Sample Acuity Tool

This acuity tool may be better described as a "best practice" due to the collage of work from all areas. The unit-based council at an HonorHealth facility in Scottsdale, Arizona, looked at how four resources could be combined to create a working document for the oncology unit. The developing tool was passed around to many day- and night-shift staff members and tweaked over three months. The tool survey was used to determine whether the group was on track. This form is interdisciplinary: Nursing assistants start the sheet, and RNs finish it before making assignments.

Here is the unit's acuity tool that staff members developed by taking several tools and creating their own, as noted in Tables 11.1 and 11.2.

TABLE 11.1   3C ACUITY TOOL: CLASSIFICATION LEVELS

	1 Point	2 Points	3 Points
Activity of Daily Living	Independent/ minimal assistance	Partial assistance with ADLs/assistance with ambulation	Complete assistance/total care/ turn q2 hours/incontinence
Assessment	Protocol-unit norm vitals and assessment	Neuro checks/drains/ remote telemetry/contin- uous pulse oximetry	Frequent vitals assessment due to medications/blood administration/ restraints/CIWA/instability/> 3 drains with I&Os/post-op
IV/Medication	Capped lines/ maintenance fluids with minimal IVPB/ IVB or pushes	PCA/epidural/multiple lines/IVPB or IVP > 3 per shift/occasional prn medications	Blood product > 2 units per shift/ IV meds > 5 per shift/frequent prn medication/insulin gtt
Nursing Intervention	Minimal nursing intervention/lab draws/pain inter- vention 1–2 times per shift	Trach suctioning q4 or less/lab draw <= q6 hr/ uncomplicated and infre- quent dressing change/ pain intervention > 3 per shift/isolation	Continuous bladder irrigation/ frequent drain emptying/uncon- trolled pain/new trach/frequent complex dressing change
Education/ Psychosocial	Minimal educa- tional and psycho- cial needs	Moderate educational/ psychosocial needs q4–6 hours/call light > 6 per shift approximately	Complex educational needs/1:1 care/call light > 8 per shift/new complex diagnosis/postmortem care
Chemo/High- Intensity Medication	No chemo/oral chemo 1–2 times per day	Chemotherapy infusion/ complex patient teaching regarding chemo/fever with neutropenia workup	Complex medication and chemo administration/patient at high risk for adverse reactions

Directions: Tally points for each patient, keeping in mind points are assigned by having one qualify- ing factor in the classification level. If there are multiple factors in the same category, points are not increased. Nursing has judgment to change acuity half steps (ex. E/M).

Easy: 6–8   Medium: 9–14   Hard: 15–18

TABLE 11.2 NURSING ASSESSMENT ACUITY TOOL

Rm	RN (RNs leave blank)	E M H	Chemo s/p AL	MISC...	N A T	Epi/RT	Alerts/ Prec	Div wt	VS q4	Diet	Accu √
3301						ALARM/Fall/ Conf/ Sitter/ Isolat					Ac&hs 0300 q_hr
3302						ALARM/Fall/ Conf/ Sitter/ Isolat					Ac&hs 0300 q_hr
3303						ALARM/Fall/ Conf/ Sitter/ Isolat					Ac&hs 0300 q_hr
3304						ALARM/Fall/ Conf/ Sitter/ Isolat					Ac&hs 0300 q_hr
3305						ALARM/Fall/ Conf/ Sitter/ Isolat					Ac&hs 0300 q_hr
3306						ALARM/Fall/ Conf/ Sitter/ Isolat					Ac&hs 0300 q_hr

E/M/H – Easy/Medium/Hard   N/A/T – Neutropenic/Anemic/Thrombocytopenic   D/C – Discharge Pending   Epi/RT – Epidural/Remote Tele

Rm	Activity	Toileting	Lab Sample	Linen/Baths *Check when complete	D/C	Lab Draw	Anti-coag
3301	Ind/x1/ x2/walker/ Rest/Total	Void/Urinal Foley/BSC/ Brief/Pan	Urine BM			RN Lab	Heparin Coumadin ASA
3302	Ind/x1/ x2/walker/ Rest/Total	Void/Urinal Foley/BSC/ Brief/Pan	Urine BM			RN Lab	Heparin Coumadin ASA
3303	Ind/x1/ x2/walker/ Rest/Total	Void/Urinal Foley/BSC/ Brief/Pan	Urine BM			RN Lab	Heparin Coumadin ASA
3303	Ind/x1/ x2/walker/ Rest/Total	Void/Urinal Foley/BSC/ Brief/Pan	Urine BM			RN Lab	Heparin Coumadin ASA
3305	Ind/x1/ x2/walker/ Rest/Total	Void/Urinal Foley/BSC/ Brief/Pan	Urine BM			RN Lab	Heparin Coumadin ASA
3305	Ind/x1/ x2/walker/ Rest/Total	Void/Urinal Foley/BSC/ Brief/Pan	Urine BM			RN Lab	Heparin Coumadin ASA

E/M/H – Easy/Medium/Hard   N/A/T – Neutropenic/Anemic/Thrombocytopenic   D/C – Discharge Pending   Epi/RT – Epidural/Remote Tele

As with any change, HonorHealth measured it using this tool with staff, as noted in Figure 11.1.

Acuity Tool Survey

1. Do you use the acuity rating tool . . .

    ○ 100% of the time

    ○ 50–99% of the time

    ○ 0–49% of the time

2. Please rate the accuracy of the E/M/H scale by nursing judgment only.

    ○ Low accuracy

    ○ Medium accuracy

    ○ High accuracy

3. Please rate the accuracy of the new acuity tool.

    ○ Low accuracy

    ○ Medium accuracy

    ○ High accuracy

4. Do you prefer . . .

    ○ Nursing judgment acuity scale

    ○ New acuity tool

5. Do you feel patient assignments are more evenly divided after the new acuity tool was implemented?

    ○ Yes

    ○ No

6. Comments: _____

   _____

FIGURE 11.1
Acuity tool survey.

Position Control/Roster Management

In earlier chapters, we discussed position control, more currently known as *roster management sheets,* which are a way to track information based on positions rather than employees for all the jobs within your unit or department. Position control also gives maximum flexibility for the distribution of FTEs (full-time equivalents) and allows you to see all your staff. Here, you can fully or partially assign multiple people to a single position or partially appoint incumbents to various positions (job sharing).

Typically, a position control sheet will show headcount, FTE amount (i.e., 0.1, 0.4, 0.8, or 1.0), position/specialty, and vacant and filled positions, and it will help you quickly compare what you have with what you need. This will assist you in taking a proactive approach—you won't be the reason you are "behind," whether in hiring or staffing, because you can focus your strategy on whom you need to hire next.

Figure 11.2 is an example of a position control sheet you may use or modify for your unit. This document is best created as an Excel spreadsheet.

Staff Involvement in Development

How do you elicit input from staff members about their schedule? If you have not considered engaging their input, make yourself accessible to them. In addition to the help you will get from your staff, their input will support the source of evidence for Magnet® documentation that wants to see organizations demonstrate how nurse leaders and clinical nurses advocate for resources to support nursing unit and organizational goals. Here, you can provide evidence that advocacy by a clinical nurse(s) resulted in allocating resources to support a nursing unit goal.

EMP No	Last Name	First Name	Certification	JOB CODE	FTE	Days	Nights	Total FTE
1111	Mensik	Jennifer	chem o	RN	1.00	1	0.00	
					RN Subtotal	1.00	0.00	0.00
					UAP Subtotal	0.00	0.00	0.00
					US Subtotal	0.00	0.00	0.00
					Grand Total	1.00	0.00	1.00

	D	N	FTE
Actual	0.00	0.00	0.00
Budget	0.00	0.00	0.00

Total budgeted FTEs	0.00
Actual Total vs Budget	0.00

FIGURE 11.2

A sample position control sheet.

> **TIP**
>
> *Being the manager does not mean you have to know all the answers. Being a leader means you engage others to identify issues and come to a solution together. If you and your staff developed the framework for scheduling and staffing, your staff will own it just as you do.*

Nursing Productivity Committee/Shared Leadership Staffing Committees

To get staff input, form a shared leadership council to assist with staffing, productivity, and resource issues. After you have created your committee, what do you cover, what do you talk about, and how do you get started?

For this book, the following steps serve as a pathway to an evidence-based decision-making style that is shared by staff and management (Lugo & Peck, 2008):

1. Develop the shared governance team and define the problem.

2. Find, interpret, and utilize research to guide decision-making.

3. Develop a strategy to improve the reassignment experience, support nurses, and provide high-quality patient care.

4. Implement recommendations.

5. Evaluate and monitor the revised program.

Many aspects of evidence needed for ANCC Magnet recognition, in which you demonstrate an excellent nursing work environment, come through a shared governance or professional governance structure. Note that councils and committees have all sorts of names in the literature but usually have the same functions and purposes. Incorporating staff input through committees enhances staff engagement and can help you on your Magnet journey.

Staff Buy-In

To implement something unique, innovative, or different, understand the culture and work with staff members to get their buy-in first. Remember, culture is formed from the bottom up in an organization. Your followers will only follow a leader in the direction they want to go. Start by setting up a vision that staff members want to be part of and persuade them to share ownership of that vision with you. Only together can you change the culture, and you will be innovative by changing your culture.

Shared leadership or staff-based committees often make two fatal mistakes: The manager talks and makes all the decisions, or the manager lets staff make all the decisions without "guardrails." *Guardrails* are rules that staff members cannot cross or break but have the flexibility to work within. Staff nurses may distrust shared leadership initiatives because of negative experiences when upper management changed or did not approve committee decisions.

Guardrails allow you to communicate nonnegotiable boundaries up front, so staff will only bring forward a recommendation that falls within those boundaries. Another benefit of guardrails is that you do not have to tell your staff members "no" after they have spent much time and energy working on a solution.

Another reason staff may not buy into the process is because managers on or outside the committee need to listen to staff. You do not need to listen and jump. However, listen and let them know you are listening. Thank them for their thoughts and input. It is OK to say you need time to research an issue and will get back to them later. It is also OK to reinforce a guardrail and explain the reason as long as it makes sense.

Staff members may not buy into the process because they fail to see improvement or change based on their decisions or evaluations. For instance, you collect data on their satisfaction with staffing and floating. You might display the results yet do nothing to address issues or tell them you heard their frustration. If so, your staff will be wary of your commitment to listening and changing. You must buy into the process to expect your staff to.

Shared Governance Impact on Scheduling

Samantha, a new graduate nurse on a telemetry floor, knew that her request for time off on Thanksgiving would be turned down at most hospitals. However, her organization had an established shared governance program that had relegated one of the most significant issues in a nurse's personal life—scheduling—to the unit level. A small group of staff nurses in each patient care unit was in charge of staffing and scheduling for their respective units. These self-schedulers had years of experience juggling timetables, so Samantha felt confident that her request would be honored.

Nursing shared governance is an organizational innovation by nurse managers that gives staff nurses legitimate control over their practice and extends their influence into areas previously controlled only by managers (Hess, 1994). The importance of self-governance to nurses' professional and personal lives is so great that some have erroneously equated the handoff of this function to shared governance itself. A state governor-initiated program to fund innovative hospital-based solutions during a cyclical nursing shortage in the 1980s gave more than $100,000 to a hospital with a shared governance proposal that was little more than a unit-based self-scheduling program. Scheduling has always been a monkey on managers' backs, and staff nurses who can crank out the perfect schedule are proud of their work. Coupled with recent state initiatives mandating hospital staffing levels, scheduling might be the most critical aspect of a nurse's hospital life.

A few weeks later, the November unit schedule, which included Thanksgiving, was posted. Samantha was working the entire weekend. What went wrong?

The three nurses who cranked out the unit schedule had been doing the job for about 10 years. Comfortable with the task, they used a formula that respected staffing levels but not always personal requests—especially those of new nurses. The schedulers were neither elected nor appointed. They had just been doing the schedule for as long as anyone could remember. So, if you are working in a shared governance organization with self-scheduling, remember to find out precisely what that means. Has this responsibility been delegated to a rotating group of staff nurses who will act responsibly and equitably in devising schedules that are in everyone's best interests? Or has the process been swapped out from managers who might have served bureaucratically for the organization's good to a group of nurses acting autocratically in their own best interests?

Shared governance has extended staff nurse participation in staffing and scheduling, once the responsibilities of only those in management. Successful unit-based self-scheduling is a process that empowers its participants to share control over staffing. Rotating responsibilities for scheduling among staff can ensure that everyone gets a turn at this critical function, provides incentives for acting appropriately, and generates equitable schedules. Without nurses, patients cannot receive care. Without fair schedules, hospitals cannot retain nurses. Self-scheduling has a long history now of addressing both needs.

–Robert G. Hess Jr., PhD, RN, FAAN

Staffing Plans

A *staffing plan* is a unit- and shift-specific plan that sets nurse staffing levels based on patient acuity and needs at any given time, available support staff, technology, the care delivery model, and other aspects covered in this book. In your state, staffing plans may be a legal requirement for a hospital. Staffing plans are a way to communicate specifics about how you will staff and schedule.

If you have a shared leadership committee, this group usually will write the staffing plan. If not, managers will write it, hopefully with staff input. The chief nurse executive, as the highest-level nurse in the hospital, will usually need to sign off on the plan because they are accountable and responsible for its correct implementation.

NOTE

Patient CareLink (PCL) is a healthcare quality and transparency collaborative that started with the Massachusetts Hospital Association (MHA) and Massachusetts Organization of Nurse Executives (MONE) and has now expanded to other organizations, including the Hospital Association of Rhode Island (HARI). Massachusetts is the first state to publicly report staffing plans for patients and families to review. To see actual staffing plans from various hospitals, visit the PCL website at https://www. patientcarelink.org/healthcare-provider-data/hospital-data/staffing-plans-reports/ faqs-about-staffing-plans.

Resource Management Committee Agenda

A *resource management committee* is an organized forum that supports optimal staffing and scheduling. The committee model ensures collaboration among nursing departments in addition to efficiency, consistency, and fairness when managing staff schedules. Nurse managers routinely meet every week to discuss staffing needs and surpluses. Standing agenda items that meet the organization's unique needs should be identified and addressed at each meeting. Typical agenda items include:

- Unit vacancy rates
- Unit productivity and staffing needs
- Staff cancellations
    a. Cross-training opportunities available for staff members to maintain their hours
    b. Order of cancellation of staff (in the event of low census)
- Casual labor (travel and registry nurses)
    a. Timing the use of casual labor to match census fluctuations
    b. Contracts that are ending or travel nurses who can be moved to another unit

- Per diem staff (opportunities to block schedule on units with higher vacancy rates)

- Staffing incentives for units with high vacancy rates

- Holiday schedules

- Self-scheduling guidelines

- Patient throughput issues as they relate to adequate staffing

One of the challenges to effectively managing nursing resources is nursing leadership participation. Managers in all nursing areas must be committed to the process and meeting attendance. Scheduling meetings on the same day and time each week can be helpful for nurse managers in planning their workloads.

–Michelle Winters, MBA, BSN, RN

Making Meaningful Changes to Processes

The difficulty in change lies with more than individuals. Change may impact roles, expectations, adoption of new standards of practice, and incorporation of additional responsibilities with unknown results (Wang et al., 2006). To facilitate a large change, ensure integration of the old and new processes, and, most importantly, include motivating your staff to continue to participate in designing, rolling out, measuring, and evaluating the change. Everyone should change on a unit, not just the manager. If staff feel that this was a top-down decision and change, successful implementation will be a challenge. This is where that vision really can help!

Measuring Your Change

You will understand your outcomes through measurement. Have you heard the saying "garbage in, garbage out"? What you decide to measure is very important to getting the best outcomes. If your measures and the associated data are bad (garbage in), then your subsequent evaluation and outcomes (garbage out) will be bad. As you present your data, they will not support your best argument and may be called out, to your dismay, in a meeting.

Everything you do—pilots, changes, your care delivery model—will be scrutinized by your staff, your boss, and their boss. Think of your unit as your own business. Analyze the value of what you plan to do. Think of these factors in creating your business case. Remember, the more quantifiable your measures, the better. And when you present your data, place your "soft, fuzzy, feel-good" info into a case study or real-life example, not just a generic bullet-point list. Doing so can impact those in your audience who are wired more to appreciate and understand its value.

Ask these questions when considering what to measure to demonstrate outcomes:

- Are there financial implications? Costs? Savings? Are you adding more staff?

- What are the equipment or technology needs?

- Is there a return on investment (ROI)? If so, when will the ROI materialize?

- What is the impact on quality measures, such as core measures and patient satisfaction? If you add staff, will improvements in these areas offset the cost?

- Will the change in your care delivery model significantly impact the length of stay? Are there patients to backfill the beds on your unit that are now more available?

- What are the benefits to staff? Patients? The community?

- What are your hospital administrators measuring and most concerned with? Does your change have a positive impact on that?

- Can you tie this back to your organization's overall or nursing-specific strategic plan?

Remember this: To determine your return on investment, you must understand how insurers pay your hospital. The three types of payment are charges or percentage of charges, per diem (flat fee per day), and per discharge (one payment for a patient based on the Diagnostic Related Group [DRG], regardless of services used or length of stay). If a large percentage of your organization's reimbursement still comes from charges, percentage of charges, or per diem, reducing the length of stay essentially reduces the payment. Payment per discharge, regardless of utilization, is where a decreased length of stay will financially benefit you and your organization. If you want to increase your staffing levels and believe that will reduce the length of stay, how you get paid may impact the result. However, remember, payment and payer should only drive how you provide care.

Measuring your change is vital. You will have no data to support your efforts if you do not have quantifiable outcomes. As hospital finances become tighter, changes with measurable outcomes and data will help to obtain the needed resources.

Staffing Application to Practice

Applying staffing principles to practice requires insight and knowledge regarding organizational staffing practices at the unit and the more global levels. One must know the care delivery model, understand how to translate staffing outcomes into financial conversations, and be alert to concerns arising from the trended data. Understanding the implications of staffing variances will enhance the opportunity to address and mitigate the unintended consequences of low or less-than-optimal staffing.

An example is one organization's use of staffing data to promote organizational improvements and optimal staffing. The organization uses a blended approach to staff modeling. Hours per patient day (HPPD) calculations provide the infrastructure for core staffing on each unit. In addition, a patient classification system (PCS) is used to identify the nursing workload for each shift in both a prospective and retrospective manner. Staffing for each shift is based on the PCS staffing forecaster. Retrospectively, there is a focus on meeting patient needs by assessing the recommended and actual staffing. The difference is considered the staffing variance.

Concerns emerged that units were consistently understaffed due to lack of available workers. Collected data demonstrated that over one year, the staffing variance of recommended to actual staffing had been trending into increasing negative numbers. Further data related to quality, safety, and service trends were also evaluated during this period. The results showed that when actual staffing was –3% or more, there was an increase in patient complaints, employee injuries, and nursing turnover. In addition, there was an associated decrease in nurse satisfaction.

These data points were presented to organizational leadership with conversations about the cost of turnover, downstream costs of employee-related injuries, expenses associated with patient satisfaction, and business strategies designed to attract patients. This data resulted in an immediate release of nursing FTEs for hiring. In addition, assessments of metrics related to quality, safety, service, and staffing continue. At the unit level, monthly reporting of recommended to actual staffing trends is evaluated with action plans created when units begin to experience a trend of negative staffing variances of –3% or greater.

–Kathleen M. Matson, MHA, MSN, RN, NE-BC

Evaluating Your Change

It is essential to understand how data will be used. Now that you have outcomes to your measures, what is the "so what?" What you find exciting or data you can collect to report has to mean something to someone besides you. When looking at your data, ask yourself "so what?" now that you have collected it. Consider the following:

- What do you do with it?
- What is the next step?

- Do you need more data?

- Did the data support why you are doing something?

- Is the data worth continuing to collect?

If you are a Magnet® facility or on the Magnet journey, remember the sources of evidence. A "so what" in the Magnet journey is that you must provide much evidence. You will, for example, have to show how you used trended data to formulate your staffing plan and allocate the necessary resources.

We have discussed staffing and shared leadership committees. You need to work with this group to make your change happen. You gave them a vision for the change but worked with them on the process. They are now owners with you.

Sample Scheduling Process Flow

As mentioned previously, having an utterly fair scheduling process may be difficult. However, this section provides a process calendar that demonstrates how to start a scheduling process, uses group sign-up for shifts, and provides options for how long to give individuals to complete tasks in each part of the scheduling process.

Here is what occurs during the various weeks of the scheduling process (see Figure 11.3):

- **Week "0":** Scheduling specialists evaluate core staffing or staffing to meet minimum requirements.

- **Week 1:** Unit leadership and staffing specialists readjust staffing core numbers if needed and mark off those whose vacation and education have been preapproved.

- **Weeks 2–4:** Schedule opens for staff to self-schedule. Note that the schedule opens for predetermined groupings at different times, so who gets to sign up first rotates as well. This also decreases the burden on the system to handle everyone trying to get into the system simultaneously.

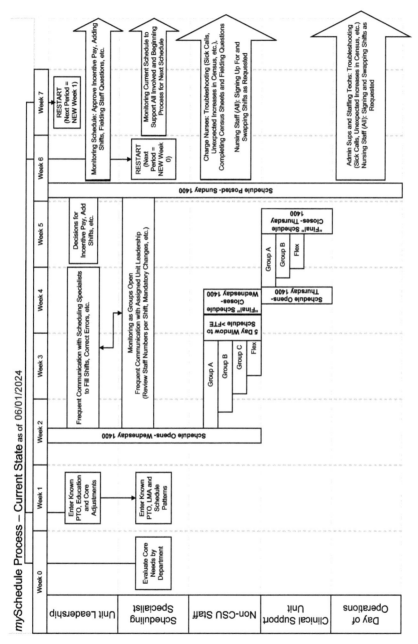

FIGURE 11.3

A sample of schedule tasks by week.

- **Week 5:** Clinical support unit, or float/per diem staff, can sign up ahead for any openings available after all floor staff have scheduled and met their FTE. A decision for incentive shifts may occur during this week, depending on how many open shifts are still available before the day of operations. In partnership with unit leaders, scheduling specialists monitor and adjust the process the entire time.

- **Week 6:** Note that in week 6, a new week "0" starts all over again, and week 7 starts a new week 1. In the other weeks, the activities in weeks 6 and 7 depend on your role in the overall process. However, because the schedule has gone live, you might monitor the day of operations changes, fill in sick calls, add incentive shifts, and perform other troubleshooting activities.

Summary

- Use shared governance as a method of staff engagement for staffing and scheduling.

- Understand the role of the manager and the role of staff on a shared governance committee.

- When determining measurements and collecting data, remember, "garbage in, garbage out."

- Use resources available online for help from states across the country.

- Make sure you pull in all data and track it to advocate for the necessary resources.

References

Hess, R. G. Jr. (1994). Shared governance: Innovation or imitation? *Nursing Economic$, 12*(1), 28–34.

Lugo, N. R., & Peck, H. (2008). Developing a shared-governance strategy to address floating. *Nursing Management, 39*(11), 8–16. https://doi.org/10.1097/01.NUMA.0000340812.75528.77

Wang, M. C., Hyun, J. K., Harrison, M. I., Shortell, S. M., & Fraser, I. (2006). Redesigning health systems for quality: Lessons from emerging practices. *Journal on Quality and Patient Safety, 32*(11), 599–611. https://doi.org/10.1016/s1553-7250(06)32078-8

Epilogue

Congratulations on finishing this book! We know how busy you are! Managing both a professional and personal life as a nurse manager is not easy. Reading a book to improve your knowledge, your skills, and your ability as a manager is not an easy thing to fit into your schedule, but you did it. We hope you learned many things that will help you in your role as a nurse manager. And most importantly, we hope you experienced a paradigm shift in thinking.

We'd like to highlight a few important concepts to take away from this book:

Start with understanding your unit's care delivery model. Understand and standardize your care delivery model, because it has a major impact on your staffing. Your unit's staffing should be in harmony with your care delivery model. If you have RNs and LPNs and NAPs, but you have a primary care delivery model, guess what? That doesn't work. Also, be sure to have one consistent care delivery model each shift, each day. Staff need to know that they will always have a primary care or a team-based delivery model (or whatever you decide) each day they come in. This decreases confusion and improves the ease of your staffing.

Maximize the capacity and capabilities of your nursing workforce. A nurse is not a nurse is not a nurse! You need to know and understand the scope of practice for all the different staff you have. You must know them all and use them to make your staffing easier and your quality of care better. Remember, create innovations, not workarounds!

Analyze and allow everyone to fully practice. Many other professionals impact your unit and staffing, and you must understand the scope and role of all individuals who may care for patients on your unit. Also, you need to ensure that your nursing staff understands the roles and that you and other managers have delineated those roles for everyone. In addition, don't be afraid to utilize other disciplines to their full potential, ability, and scope to provide patient care.

Recognize and manage variability. While it may be easy to blame your unit's issues on the fact that your patients are different, don't! You need to assess and know your variability. Remember, eliminate your artificial variability and manage the natural variability.

Target technology that improves staffing and outcomes. While some might not agree, technology such as clinical decision support systems can make nurses more efficient. Technology is just a piece of innovation, but it has significant impacts on patient safety and quality. When implementing new technology or just getting your staff to embrace the technology you have, don't forget the power of role-modeling the technology to others in a patient-centered manner.

Tie all your pieces together. It's always important to remember that a good idea at the wrong time ends up being a bad idea! Timing is important in successful adoption of change. If something didn't work before, consider trying it again. As you go forward in doing something innovative and different, make sure you create a shared vision for change with your staff. Your staff buy-in is vital to your success.

Just as we have shared our experiences and many others' great experiences in this book, we hope you do the same. As you learn what not to do, or you create a great solution to your staffing and scheduling process, we hope you communicate it, whether by writing it up for a journal or presenting it with your colleagues at a local, state, or national conference. Remember, we all learn from each other. Just as we need to share what works, we also need to share what doesn't. It's all about learning, not about what's wrong or right.

In closing, again, we hope you have learned something, we hope you think differently about staffing, and we hope that maybe your paradigm shifted as it relates to staffing and scheduling!

Index

Note: Page references noted with an *f* are figures; page references noted with a *t* are tables.

A

Academy of Medical-Surgical Nurses (AMSN), 33

Accountable Care Organizations (ACOs), 25, 26, 27, 233

accuracy of clinical decision support (CDS), 166

activity-based method, 38–40

acuity
  quantifying, 39, 185
  sample acuity tool, 246–250

admissions
  assessments, 218
  scheduling, 145, 146

advanced practice registered nurses (APRNs), 88, 111–113. *See also* nursing

Affordable Care Act of 2010, 169, 233

Agency for Healthcare Research and Quality (AHRQ), 21

agendas, resource management committee, 257–258

aging workforce, 100

allocation, artificial variability, 145–148

allowance time, 187

ambulatory care, 235–237

American Association of Critical-Care Nurses (AACN), 33

American Case Management Association (ACMA), 124

American Nurses Association (ANA), 33
  Code of Ethics, 15, 163
  definition of nursing, 6
  definition of nursing process, 7–9
  Membership Assembly, 160
  professional performance, 7*t*
  Scope and Standards of Practice, 91–92
  Social Policy Statement, 16
  standards of practice, 5*t*, 7

American Nurses Credentialing Center (ANCC), 214

S